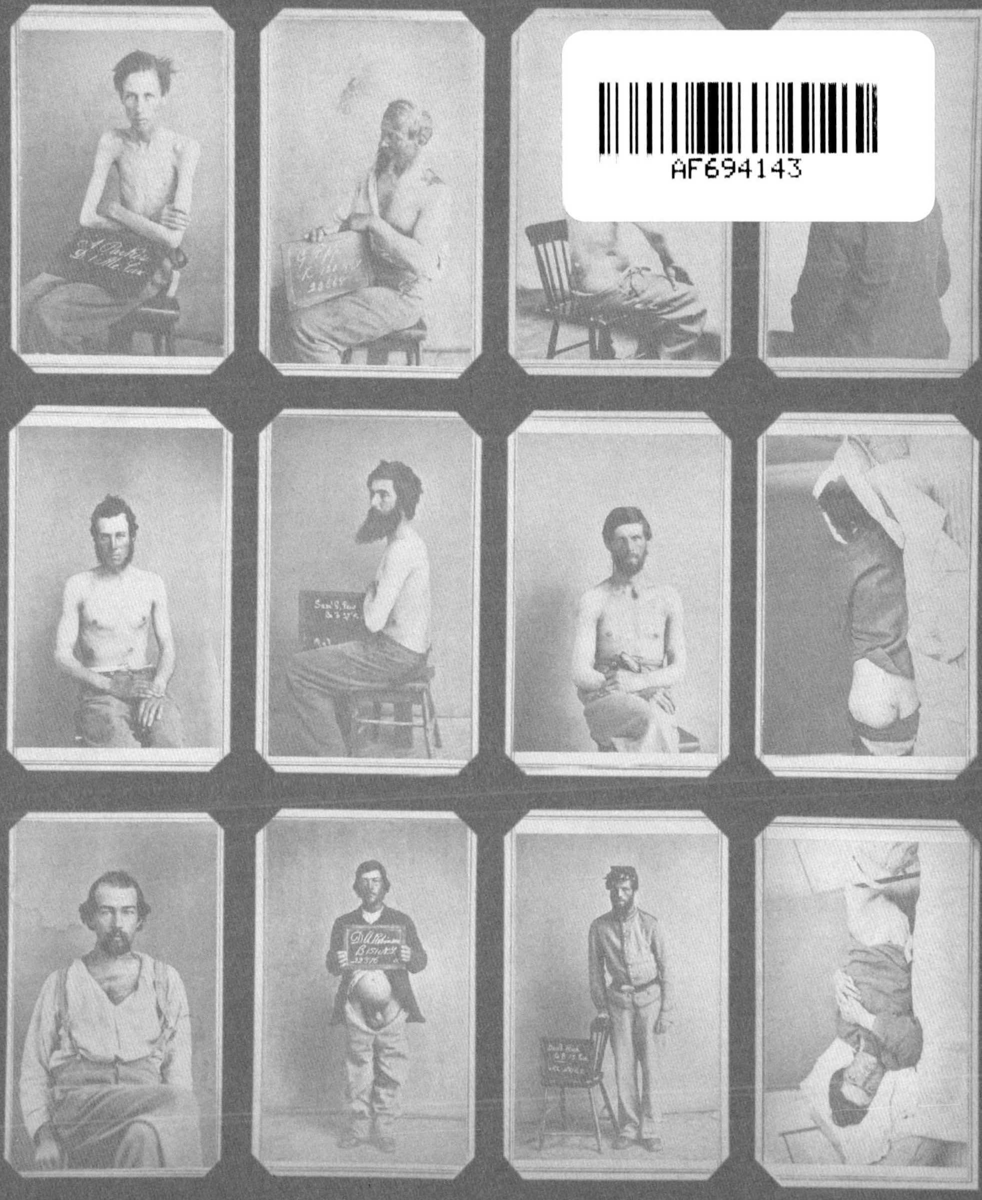

428

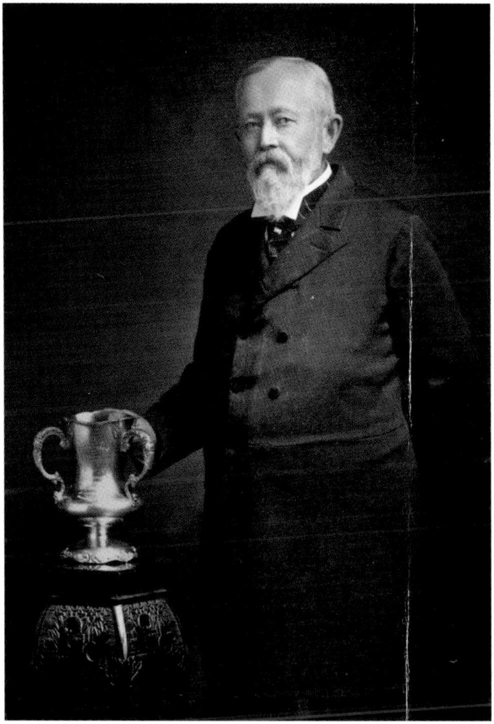

"I look back at my life at Washington with regrets that it could not last always."

REED
BROCKWAY
BONTECOU
1824 1907

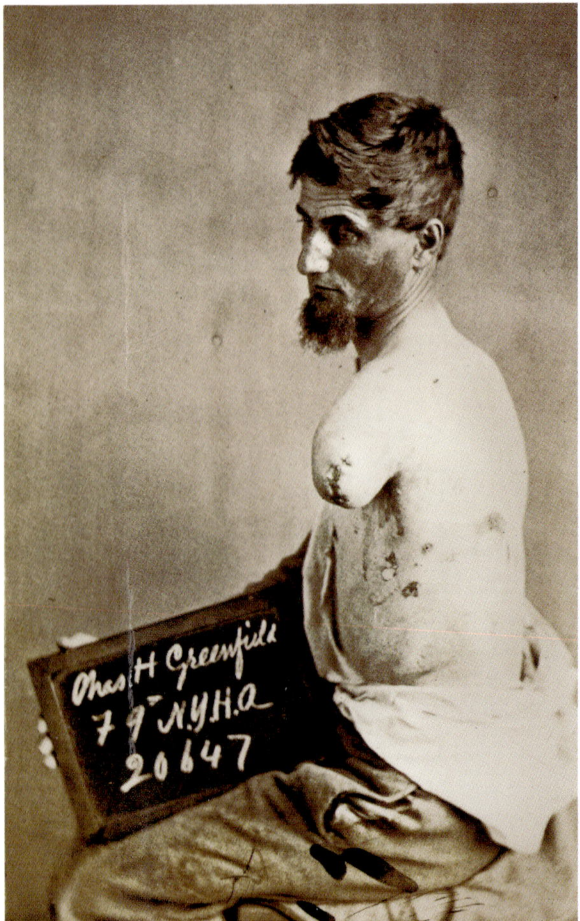
Chas H Greenfield
7th N.Y.H.A
20647

SHOOTING SOLDIERS

CIVIL WAR MEDICAL PHOTOGRAPHY BY

REED B. BONTECOU, MD

BOOK ONE: WOUNDED SOLDIERS IDENTIFIED
101 REGIMENTS FROM THE HAREWOOD HOSPITAL ALBUM

STANLEY B. BURNS, M.D.
CLINICAL PROFESSOR OF MEDICINE & PSYCHIATRY
NEW YORK UNIVERSITY LANGONE MEDICAL CENTER

FOREWORD BY MICHAEL RHODE
CHIEF ARCHIVIST, NATIONAL MUSEUM OF HEALTH & MEDICINE

BURNS ARCHIVE PRESS

Published by The Burns Archive Press, an imprint of The Burns Archive,
New York, New York
ISBN 13 978-1-936002-05-4
ISBN 10 1-936002-05-1

Library of Congress Cataloging-in-Publication Data:
Burns, Stanley B.
Shooting Soldiers, Civil War Medical Photography by Reed B. Bontecou, MD,
1. Photographic--History 2. Civil War--History 3. Medical--History 4. Medical--Photography 5. Reed B. Bontecou, MD 6. Cultural History 7. Stanley B. Burns--Photographic Collections

BURNS ARCHIVE PRESS

AUTHOR & PUBLISHER: STANLEY B. BURNS, MD, FACS
PRODUCTION & DESIGN: LISSA RIVERA
TEXT & COPY EDITOR: LESLIE HODGKINS
RESEARCH ASSISTANTS: SARAH SIMMS, LISSA RIVERA, ALICE DANA
HISTORIC PHOTOGRAPHS: © STANLEY B. BURNS, MD & THE BURNS ARCHIVE

THIS BOOK IS THE SECOND IN A SERIES OF CATALOGUES OF THE BURNS COLLECTION

FRONT COVER: J.E. JOLIFF, 116TH PENNSLYVANIA, GUN SHOT WOUND, LEFT LEG. WOUNDED AT PETERSBURG APRIL 6, 1865. DISCHARGED JULY 12, 1865.

BACK COVER: H. PARQUETTE, 1ST NEW HAMPSHIRE, HEAVY ARTILLARY,FORT SLOCUM SEPTEMBER 14, 1864, ACCIDENTAL EXPLOSION OF SHELL TEALE'S AMPUTATION OF LEGS BY BONTECOU. TRANFERRED TO MANCHESTER USA GEN'l HOSP MAY 17TH 1865.

FRONTISPIECE: CHARLES H. GREENFIELD, 79TH NEW YORK, HA, PETERSBURG, APRIL 2, 1865, AMPUTATION OF LEFT ARM ON FIELD, DISCHARGED JULY 9 1865.

TITLE PAGE: DR. BONTECOU HONORED AT A SPECIAL DINNER OF THE RENSSELAER COUNTY MEDICAL SOCIETY PRESENTED WITH A SILVER CUP FOR HIS CONTRIBUTIONS TO MEDICINE, NOVEMBER 18, 1903.

CONTENTS

FOREWORD

I've known Dr. Stanley Burns for twenty-five years and have watched with appreciation as he built an excellent collection of photographs of medical subjects and history. Dr. Burns, an ophthalmologist by training, has demonstrated a wide range of interests in his collecting, but one subject that he continues to return to is the Civil War. His focus has been on Dr. Reed Bontecou, whose association with the Army Medical Museum spanned from 1862 during the Civil War until at least 1894 when he wrote in for diagnostic help on a difficult case. Bontecou was by no means the only photographer working with the Museum. On our staff was professional photographer William Bell, who had other photographers assisting him. Contributors such as Dr. James Armsby of the Army's Ira Harris General Hospital in Albany, New York also provided hundreds of photographs. The contributions of Bontecou and Armsby, among scores of others, were numbered as 'Contributed Photographs' in the Museum's collection, and then frequently copied and published as 'Surgical Photographs' or 'Photographs of Surgical Cases and Specimens' to be distributed to medical professionals.

One of the difficulties of untangling the history of these pictures has been the long amount of time since they were taken and the revival of interest in them. In 1986, the photographs had then recently been returned to the Museum's control from another division of the pathology institute that grew out of, and ultimately took over, the Museum. The collections were all intermingled and no inventory existed. Computer technology was still primitive, and the main way to track these images was to use an 1876 index card system. These index cards reveal that about half of the collection of Contributed Photographs is now missing. Many of the images taken by Dr. Bontecou were returned to his son Dr. R.B. Bontecou Jr. in March 1915 by Museum pathologist Dr. Daniel S. Lamb. Lamb had worked at the Museum since the Civil War, when he was a hospital steward. He stayed there through earning his medical degree, volunteered at Freedmen's Hospital when not busy at the Museum, and at the end of his career was reorganizing the Museum's photographs. Unfortunately for us, that meant he frequently disposed of them and hundreds of glass plate negatives of Civil War images were discarded as broken or uninteresting. Fortunately for everyone though, Dr. Burns' interest in these photographs has led him to track down, preserve and publicize a significant amount of them.

It's a great pleasure to see these images in print. Even I have never seen most of them. In these days of digital copies, it is hard to imagine how difficult it was to take a clean piece of glass, coat it with a photographic emulsion and let it dry in the dark, expose it in sunlight (since there was no flash photography), develop the plate in the dark, and then print the picture by laying a negative on a piece of photographic paper in the sunlight. The photographic paper would then be bathed in a chemical bath in the dark to permanently fix the image. And that was the new, improved process! Dr. Burns has done the medical and photographic history communities a great service by rescuing and making these images available again, and I know this book will be a valuable addition to many libraries.

Michael Rhode
Chief Archivist, Otis Historical Archives
National Museum of Health and Medicine

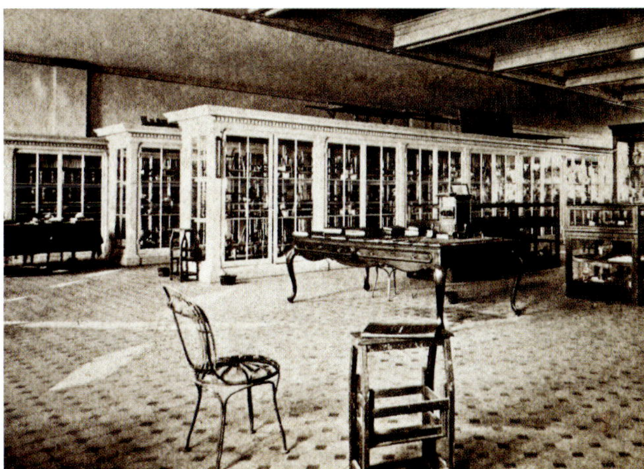

ARMY MEDICAL MUSEUM, CIRCA, 1868.

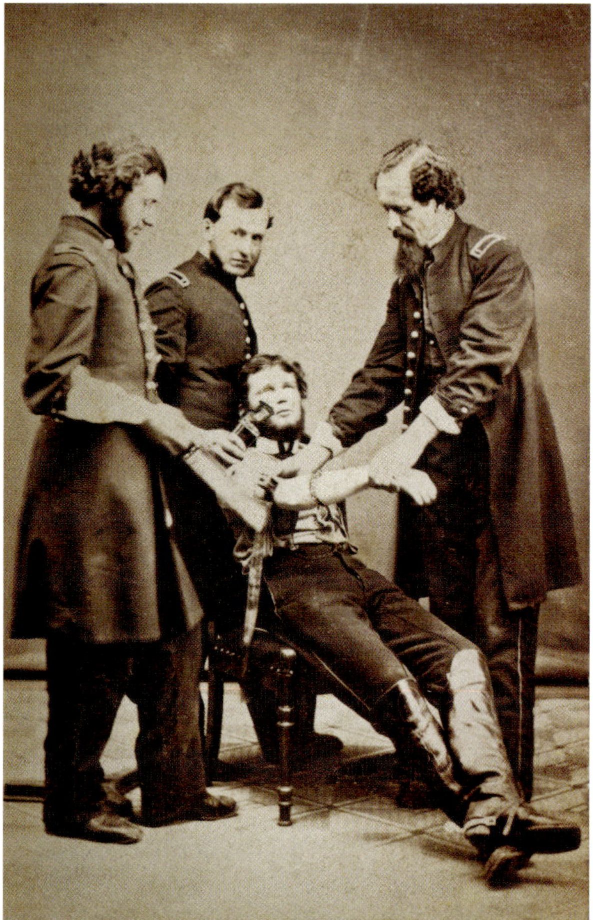

IN FIELD HOSPITALS, ARM AMPUTATIONS WERE SOMETIMES PERFORMED WITH THE PATIENT SEATED IN A CHAIR. ONE PHYSICIAN HOLDS THE SAW, ANOTHER A BOTTLE OF ETHER FOR AMPUTATION. (POSED VIEW). SIGNED VERSO S. BAIRD WOLFF, MD., POST SURGEON WITH LOGO OF D. P. BARR, ARMY PHOTOGRAPHER, PADUCAH KY., CDV, 1864.

PREFACE

I have always been fascinated with the human condition. The depth of "Man's inhumanity to his fellow Man" has both intrigued and disturbed me. As an ophthalmologist, a visual specialist and a photo historian, I learned that most people think in pictures and that perhaps creating visual essays showing the results of hatred, slavery, abuse and war would bring greater awareness to the true nature of the phenomena and change some opinions. Censorship of war images has until lately been one of the critical programs of warring nations. Pictures of a country's dead and severely wounded servicemen are usually withheld from the public until long after the conflict. Censorship can be a two edged sword with unintended consequences.

As a child I became interested in history. While doing research, in 1956, as a freshman at Brooklyn College I discovered in the library stacks Francis Miller's ten volume, *The Photographic History of the Civil War*. I was thrilled to see Mathew Brady's images and felt transported back in time to the reality of the war. It was the first time I had seen a vintage photographic text and I was totally captivated by the images. The Civil War was special to me because while growing up in the 1940s I spent the summers in Harris, New York. Living in the house next door was Mr. Calkins, a retired farmer who would show me the guns and equipment his father used in the war and related the stories told to him. I was fascinated by the stories and handling the equipment and in 1962 I began to collect the weapons of the Civil War. I finished medical school during the Vietnam War era and In the mid 1960s I spent six years in the US Public Health Service, detailed at times as a general surgeon to the US Coast Guard on ships and helicopters doing rescues for which I received a commendation. Being a first responder to care for the severely injured became an experience that further peaked my interest in medical care for wounded serviceman. In 1975, I discovered the availability of vintage photography and began to collect images concentrating on daguerreotypes, war, postmortem, medical and ethnic images. I sold the arms collection and used the funds to buy photographs. From the start I was drawn to collecting all aspects of medical photography. The human devastation of war remains one of my main interests and I have albums of wounded soldiers from the Civil War through World War II. In 1976 I discovered the amazing pioneer work of Civil War surgeon Reed Brockway Bontecou, who documented his patients in an artistic manner that has intrigued audiences from their inception. I have his four original Civil War albums and I am pleased to share these original clinical photographs.

INTRODUCTION

A new significant chapter in Civil War history is revealed with this first exposé of the war-time clinical photographs of Reed Bontecou. Through his remarkable portraits, Bontecou created and became a legend. Walt Whitman in *Specimen Days* noted that "The real war will never get in the books." It was just too horrendous, brother killing and maiming brother in tens of thousands of episodes. Whitman served as a volunteer nurse in the war making thousands of visits to hospitals. He saw first hand the devastation the new 'minie ball' bullets did to bodies. He commented, "there were just too many stories and incidents to tell about the heroic and even ordinary men of the war." Surgeon Reed Brockway Bontecou, armed with his camera, perhaps gets closest to the individual reality of the Civil War and his photographs may refute Whitman's claim. Bontecou's photographs are the visual evidence of the real war, the bottom line of the war as it affects individuals and families. His poignant views of wounded servicemen indelibly etch the mind and help us better appreciate the sacrifice these men made to achieve the highest goal of mankind: a just and equal society for all.

The Civil War is America's *Iliad*, Homer's Greek tragedy about war. It is America's greatest universal epic with mythic proportions that have entranced historians with the magnitude of its political, personal and ideological concepts. Burial played a big role in *The Iliad* as ancient Greek culture stressed proper burial as a requirement for the soul's peaceful rest. The Civil War mimics *The Iliad* as it was a war that not only erased lives but identities as well; hundreds of thousands are buried "unknown."

This is the first volume of a series showcasing the Civil War carte de visite (CdV) photographs of Reed Brockway Bontecou, MD, Surgeon-in-Charge of Harewood U.S. Army General Hospital, Washington DC. He was responsible for pioneering and taking the largest number of photographs of wounded soldiers during the war and was the largest contributor of photographs and specimens to the Army Medical Museum and Civil War medical publications. His close-up images of surgery, anesthesia, and patients posing with their pathological specimens were unique for his time. Many photographs are of patients pre and post operation, views of patients showing the progression of specific treatments, or the various stages of diseases. After the war, he organized his photographs into albums laying them out, anatomically from head to foot wounds, and loosely alphabetically by soldier's name. The CdV album is an amazing visual document of medical aspects of war and was not equaled until fifty years later in WWI.

The album is also the pioneering effort by one physician to document war wounds and to use photography to teach physicians how to care for these wounds. Bontecou was a true innovator in clinical war photography. Many of his images are beautifully posed, elevating clinical photography to an art form.

The Surgeon General Office's publications after the war used photographs and Bontecou was the largest contributor. These noteworthy landmark publications set the standard for other nations to follow in analyzing the medical effects and efforts in war. The most significant of these volumes, the six volume *Medical & Surgical History of the War of the Rebellion* is liberally illustrated with engravings made from photographs of Bontecou's most interesting cases. None of the clinical images were published as photographs, most of these images are now reproduced photographically in this series for the first time.

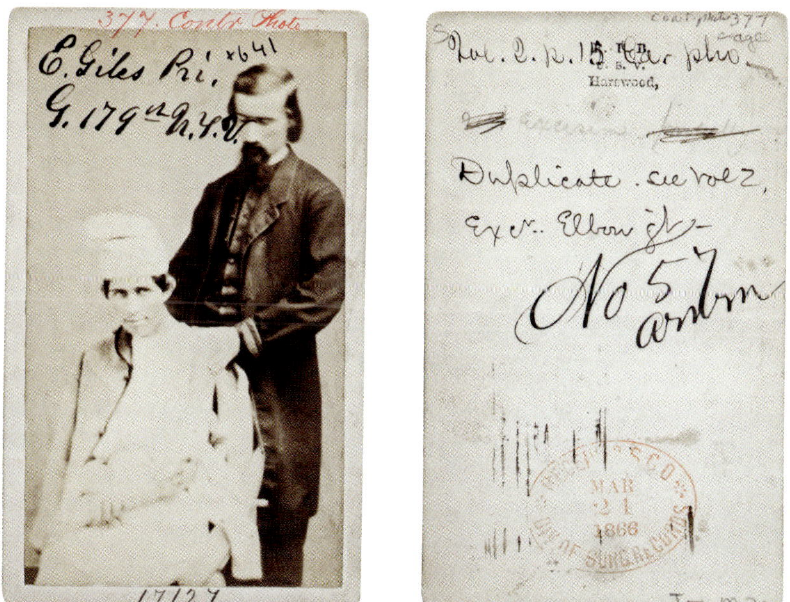

CONTRIBUTED PHOTOGRAPH WITH MARKINGS FROM THE ARMY MEDICAL MUSEUM, CDV, 1866.

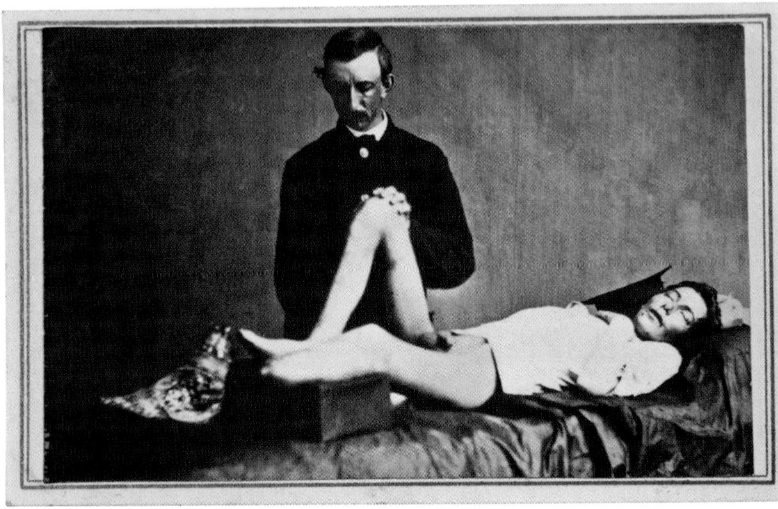

PVT. JOHN PARMENTER, CO G 67 PA, LYING UNCONCIOUS FROM ANESTHESIA ON OPERATING TABLE WITH HIS SEVERED FOOT. HOSPITAL GANGRENE NECESSITATED AMPUTATION JUNE 21, 1865. WOUNDED APRIL 3, 1865 AT AMELIA SPRINGS, VA.

Due to their historical precedence there can be no doubt that Bontecou's carte de visite album is the premier medical photograph album of the Civil War. No other large compilation of war-time clinical images exists, with over 570 images. Almost all the photos were taken during the war or immediately after in the spring of 1865. This is in distinction to copy prints made after the war by Bontecou and to those photographs taken several years later of healed wounds for pension purposes by an assortment of photographers. Many of the large (5 ½ by 7 ½ inch) clinical photographs associated with the war are copy print enlargements of Bontecou's CdVs, in most cases they are cropped versions produced after the war. The CdVs are the original full frame image and presented here as they were made. Photography connoisseurs are always looking for the original print made at the time the image was taken. These images are those rare first printing photographs and more importantly, since so few were made many of the images are unique and have never been published until now.

To place the photographs in context of their creation, a history of Bontecou's career will be presented along with a history of the various images and albums he made.

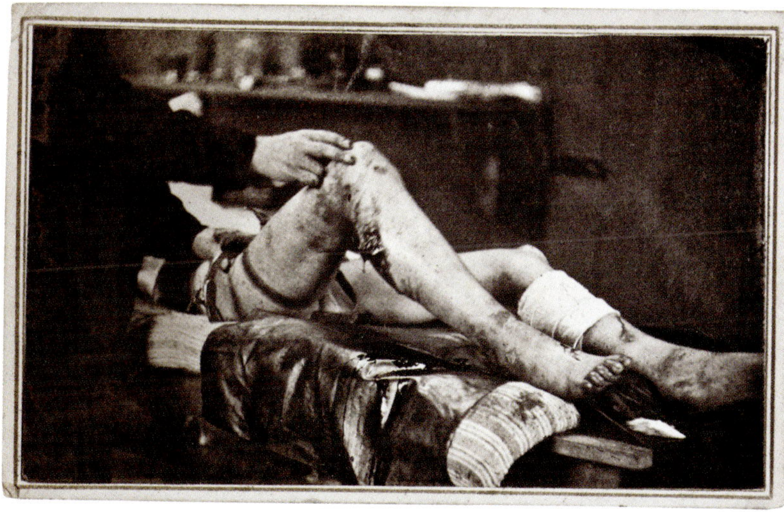

BONTECOU'S CLOSE-UP IMAGES OF PATIENTS IN OPERATING ROOMS AND OF SURGERY IN PROGRESS ARE THE EARLIEST KNOWN SUCH VIEWS. PRIOR TO AN AMPUTATION WE SEE THE TOURNIQUET ABOUT THE THIGH AND OILED CLOTH TABLE DRAPE. STERILE PRECAUTIONS WERE UNKNOWN AT THIS TIME.

A summary of the last campaigns of the war are also briefly documented. As Civil War historians are often interested in studying specific regiments, a list of the units represented is documented along with a list of the battles and the specific soldiers wounded in them. About 103 plates of soldiers from the CdV album posing with identification boards are included. and arranged by states but not numerically by unit number. Some photographs in the text are examples from Bontecou's large format albums. Also discussed are the artistic and scientific merit of the images. A presentation of the role of sacrifice and death during the Civil War era is important in helping understand the general mental state of servicemen of that era. This chapter documents some death and dying concepts in the time period and emphasizes the lack of concern of Federal government authorities for identification and proper burial of servicemen. It cannot be overemphasized that this was an American war in which we fought among ourselves. It was not fought by professional soldiers but by about 3 million citizen volunteers on American soil. The viciousness of the conflict was expected as each side was protecting their homeland, whether Petersburg, Virginia or Gettysburg, Pennsylvania.

THE ART OF THE IMAGES

Many of Dr. Bontecou's compelling artistic interpretations of war wounds are recognized as among the highest levels of photographic art. The images have a universal appeal not only as photographs but as anti war documents. They illustrate an aspect of an all-to-common universal condition – the personal results of war. The images portray men, young and old, staring at us stoically, carrying their wounds as we look and react to them through the safe distance of time. These powerful images have transfixed audiences both professional and public since their creation. We are drawn to these men because they speak a universal language of war. The fascination with Bontecou's images transcends both the historical and clinical. They are human documents. Like the poetry and prose of Walt Whitman's *Specimen Days* and Stephen Crane's fiction *The Red Badge of Courage*, the photographs are eloquent works of art that offer unflinching testimony to the suffering caused by America's bloodiest war.

The visual culture of medicine continues to intrigue audiences as the public has become accustomed to seeing vintage medical photographs in museums, galleries and online. Bontecou's photographs were originally made as medical documents of war but in about a decade they were transformed into national icons. The magnitude of the war's significance and the sacrifice by so many for political and philosophical ideals cemented the images together into a visual legacy that had to be shared with the entire nation. The Army Medical Museum (AMM) within a few years of the war's end began mounted exhibitions of the photographs around the country and published texts with the images for medical and scientific audiences.

In 1876, the United States celebrated its Centennial with a huge exposition in Philadelphia. The Army Medical Museum put many of the medical photographs on display, bringing them to general public attention. However, it must be noted that the museum staff altered the images. The genital area if exposed was covered with a fig leaf, which had been added to the negatives. This was not done in consideration of protecting the privacy of the patient but to protect the Victorian public's sensitivities. Today legal considerations preclude the display of clinical photographs, but until the early twentieth century there were few patient's privacy concerns. The soldiers whose images were on display reacted positively, they were proud of the public acknowledgement of their service. The eleven years since the war ended had elevated those that served into national heroes who had saved the Union and freed the slaves. The photographs also served as proof of disability for pension purposes as well as veteran and survivor benefits.

No written description of a wound or deformity compares to the visual representation. For all, the photographs would survive through time as iconic images of the reality of war. These clinical photographs were not perceived as private or protected documents so they enjoyed a long public life that allowed them to be viewed, interpreted and reinterpreted. Today they are commonly found in art museums.

These staged photographs are classics and are among the best of early clinical photography. The pose is determined so as to best show the patient's condition without cutting the patient himself out of the picture. Most of the images are reminiscent of Mathew Brady and other notable photographers' posing standards. As a result in many cases the images challenge some audience's concept of artistic expression because what is shown is not conventionally "beautiful." Bontecou and his photographers, like all great photographers, were masters of exposing the nature of the sitter. The sitter with wounds, disease and deformity was presented as naturally as possible. It should be noted that smiling in photographs during this early period was very rare and the subject put on his best expression. The images are portraits presenting the wounded as people, not specimens. This is in contrast to the images of AMM photographers William Bell and Edward Ward. The photographs they produced for the seven volume *Photographs of Surgical Cases and Specimens…* of clinical cases are repetitive, simplistic, nonpersonal views of servicemen. They depict, in most cases a naked soldier, or a soldier with a rolled up shirt displaying his wounds. These views may serve a clinical purpose but they do not have the power or artistry of Bontecou's images. They are not compelling views.

Over the past 30 years I have written about the advance of medical photography. The closer physicians got to understanding a disease the more attuned the photograph was to showing the basic defect. Today an image of a gene or gene sequence represents a disease. Prior medical images included close ups of the diseased part, histological/ or microscopic views, and so on. The holistic concept of a full photograph of the patient brings the individuality of the condition to how it affects that person.

Bontecou's clinical images continue to fascinate to this day as each new audience discovers them. All the prior audiences saw enlarged copy prints of the images, which were made after the war. This series presents for the first time the original full frame photographs in their original context. The National Museum of Health and Medicine's Michael Rhode, Chief Archivist at the Otis Historical Archives and J.T.H. Connor, Assistant Director, have written a comprehensive critical review of the images and their place in cultural history.

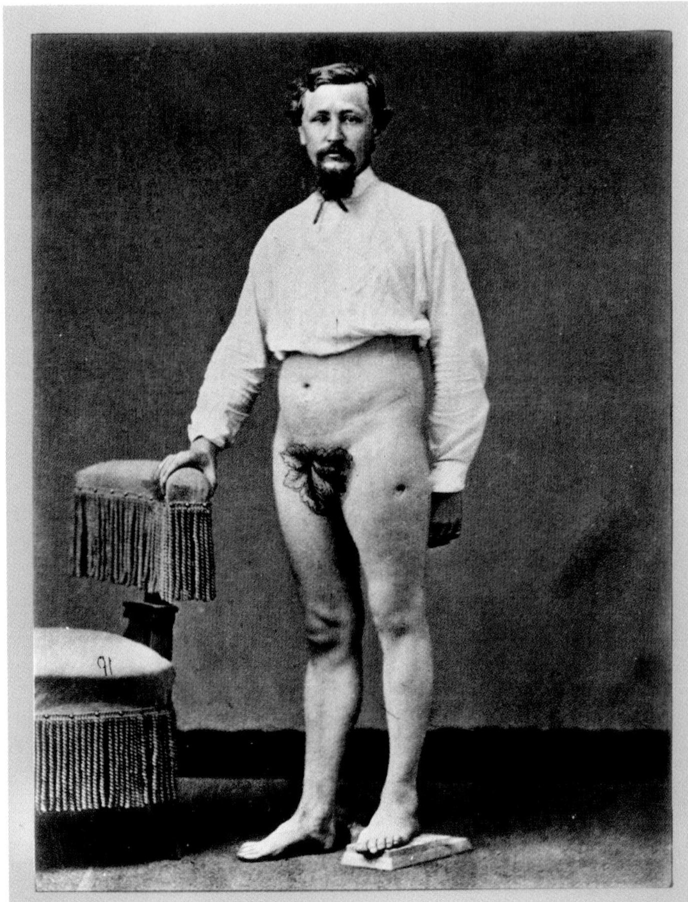

WILLIAM BELL WHO BECAME THE PHOTOGRAPHER AT THE ARMY MEDICAL MUSEUM AND WHOSE PHOTOGRAPHS WERE PUBLISHED IN A FIVE VOLUME PHOTOGRAPHIC TEXT HAS A DISTINCTIVE STYLE. HIS IMAGES MOST OFTEN DEPICT SOLDIERS STANDING OR SITTING WITH THEIR SHIRTS ROLLED UP UNDER THEM OR THEY ARE NUDE. THE IMAGES HAD AN ADDED FIG LEAF PUT IN THE NEGATIVE FOR THE 1876 US CENTENNIAL. BONTECOU'S PHOTOGRAPHS (RIGHT) ARE MORE LIKE ARTISTIC PORTRAITS, THE MEN DEPICTED IN A VARIETY OF POSES IN VARIOUS STAGES OF DRESS, MANY IN THEIR UNIFORMS.

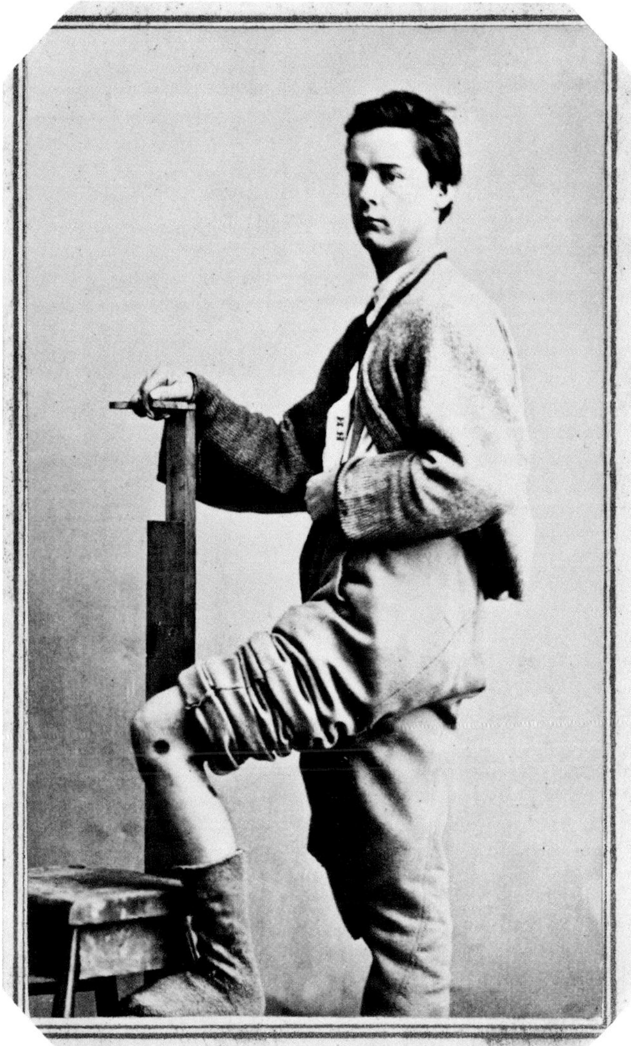

They posit that the photographers and subjects knew they were creating important lasting documents. The authors also acknowledge Bontecou's seminal role, noting: "the transformation of such specimens into national icons and symbols of political and professional unity, and development of medical photography and its significance -- coalesce in the work of Dr. Reed Bontecou." Any future clinical war photographs will be compared with these initial profound images of the Civil War.

After the war ended and while still serving at Harewood Hospital, (until June 1866), Bontecou began preparing three sets of enlarged copy print albums made from the CdVs. Aside from Bontecou's personal set in the Burns Collection there are surviving sets in both the Cornell and Yale University libraries. Cultural historians who have evaluated Bontecou's photographs in published works have analyzed them only from these post war album sets that contain the enlarged copy print 5 ½ by 7½ inch oval images. These larger images are matted on tag board and surrounded by a sepia and gold colored border 'frame.' The reactions and emotional responses of those who discover these images for themselves run an intellectual gamut. Cultural historians have described these images as romantic stamps of the era and the borders as boundaries between these wounded others and ourselves. Kathy Newman studied the photograph albums at Yale and Blair Rogers, MD the albums at Cornell University. Dr. Rogers, a plastic surgeon, was mainly interested in the head, neck and face wounds and invites the reader to study the images carefully and reflect on the emotions they elicit. Newman remarks on how the "gilded frame cannot mitigate the wastedness of his body or the raggedness of his amputated limb. [The photograph] unveils the truth of the disease (gangrene) only to discover that the horror of war…lies beneath." Other writers have been intrigued by the simplicity and power of the images.

Aside from the albums Bontecou produced himself, some of his photographs where featured in postwar photographic publications produced by the AMM and Surgeon General's Office (SGO). In 1869, George Otis, MD in the SGO, compiled a unique volume, *Photographs Contributed to the Army Medical Museum….* It contains 109 images, more than half were Bontecou's 5 ½ by 7 ½ inch prints. Otis also produced other albums from the images for use at the AMM and US Centennial. All these albums are still housed at the museum. In 1871 the five volume *Photographs of Surgical Cases and Specimens Taken at the Army Medical Museum* was completed and issued. Another two volumes were produced in the 1870s. In 1881, a unique eighth volume was created by the AMM, which contains mainly civilian images and photos related to the assassination of President Garfield that same year. Each volume contains 50 photographs. About ten of Bontecou's images appear in this series, the rest of the images were taken after the war in the AMM. The photographer for the first volume of 50 images is unknown. Photographer William Bell (1830-1910), who began work at the AMM in 1868, took most of the images from numbers 51 to 200 and Edward J. Ward, who began photographing at the AMM in 1871, took most of the rest. E.D Hudson, prosthetic maker, and surgeon Gurdon Buck, both of New York City, also contributed images. Many of the photographs were of bones and other pathological specimens. About 40 sets were produced of the first five volumes. These photographic texts were sent to army medical directors and then to American and foreign medical institutions.

Today medical photographs are private documents only for view by health care professionals. It will be some time before modern medical war imagery becomes available for scholarly scrutiny or public view. Whatever the case, future war clinical war photographs will always be compared with the amazing set of Bontecou's images. His place in the art of photography and medicine is assured. Bontecou's photographs became outdated as clinical specimens, with the discoveries related to bacteriology, wound infection and surgical sepsis. Nothing, however, can outdate the power and direct authority with which they serve as specimens of that scourge for which we have yet too have discovered an effective treatment: The scourge of war.

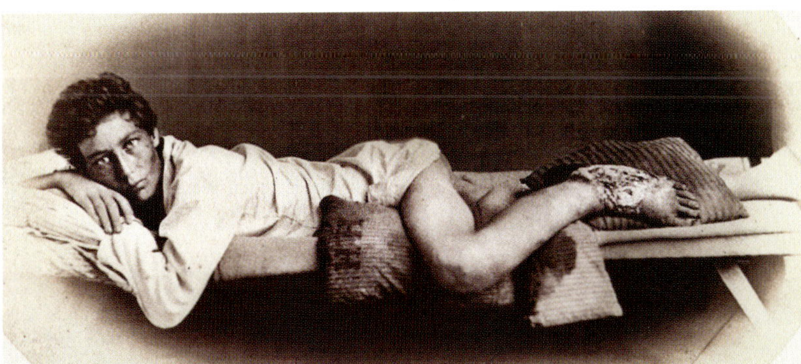

JOHN PARMENTER, CO G 67 PA, (SEE ALSO PAGE 8) PRE-OPERATIVE VIEW WITH HOSPITAL GANGRENE.

HISTORY OF THE BONTECOU PHOTOGRAPHS

The Army Medical Museum (AMM) was the greatest medical legacy of the Civil War. The museum was the brainchild of innovative, outspoken maverick US Surgeon General William Alexander Hammond, MD (1828-1900). The inadequate response of the antiquated, disorganized Federal medical units in the early battles of the war necessitated an overhaul of the system. In April 1862, Dr. Hammond was appointed surgeon general of a newly reorganized Army Medical Department. Among his far-reaching and novel proposals was the establishment of an Army Medical School as well as a medical museum. It would take 100 years for the medical school to be established but other innovations were immediately implemented. In Circular No. 5 issued June 9, 1862 Hammond outlined his plans. The goal of the medical museum was educational and specific: to improve the care of the wounded soldier, to teach physicians proper effective therapies, to study wounds, and to publish. The publication of statistical results of treatment became one of the ultimate medical achievements of the war and directly led to other countries following this methodology. Between 1870 and 1888 six elephantine sized quarto volumes, three medical and three surgical, were produced. In *The Medical and Surgical History of the War of the Rebellion (MSHWR)* almost every Union casualty is listed and statistically analyzed, as well as the results of treatment. Hundreds of personal narratives of physicians' war experience's are included.

The basic concept of the museum was the accumulation of objects and data of lasting scientific importance. It was the duty of medical officers to submit interesting specimens to the museum. At first this was interpreted as pathological specimens: body parts, wounding missiles and other paraphernalia. On January 1, 1863, less than six months after its establishment, the AMM published its first book; *Catalogue of the Army Medical Museum*. It described the 1,349 objects in the museum's collection and reiterated request for further specimens. It also clearly presented for the first time official mention of a request for photographs. A typical request contains this suggestion to the medical officers of the Army as to the forwarding of specimens to the AMM:

> "1: Specimens illustrative of surgical injuries and affections: such as----Photographic representations of extraordinary injuries, portraying the results of injuries, operations, or peculiar amputations."

Thus in 1863, collecting photographic specimens was designated a duty of Army surgeons. These photographs were labeled "contributed" and they were numbered. The carte de visite (CdV) became the most popular medium with which to document clinical cases.

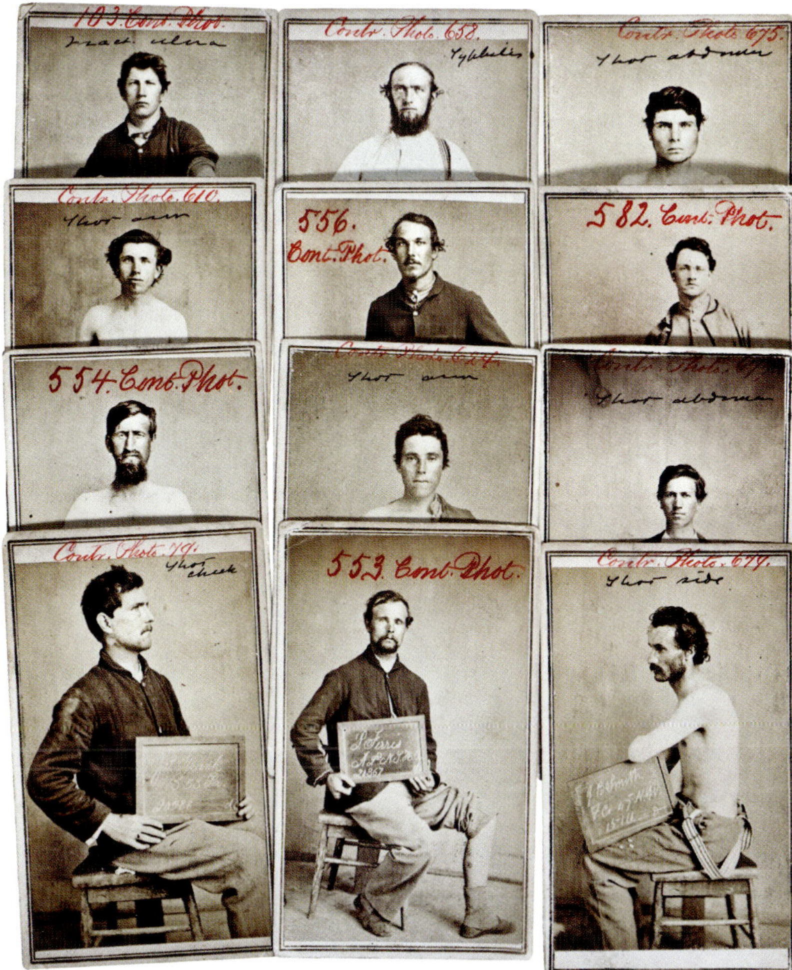

1: J. SWOYER 93RD PA, W. LIMBER 2ND NY CAV, A. SMITH 69TH NY

2: F. J. ESSELMAN 20TH MI, J. C. EGLER 2ND NY, (ILLEGIBLE NAME) 50TH PA

3: M. DECKER 6TH WI, M. KELKELLY 37TH MA, J. SEILER 208TH PA

4: J. STRUNK 53RD PA, P. FARIS 2ND NY HA, J. B. SMITH 47TH NY

Field surgeons and those actively participating in first response care were not able to photograph their patients. The slow wet plate camera, in fact, could not record actual battles as any movement resulted in a blur. At the general hospitals where patients were treated and recuperating the taking of an admitting and discharge or healed-stage photograph was realized by Reed Bontecou, MD. He is credited as the innovator of these war related clinical photographs. Surgeon J. Cooper McKee of Lincoln General Hospital in Washington, and J.H. Armsby of Ira Harris General Hospital in Albany, New York, and physicians at the Fredericksburg General Hospital also prepared CdV photographs of wounded soldiers at the end of the war and presented their albums to the AMM. These collections are still in the museum. By 1869, about 900 CdV's were in the AMM collection, housed in four volumes. Many of these photographs were used to make engravings for the MSHWR and were so marked on the CdV. During the early twentieth century the first 898 of the CdV photographs were dispersed by museum personnel. The AMM has numbers 899 through 4355. The later numbers were various size prints, 3 by 5 inch and larger and were contributed mainly in the late 1800s. Earlier in the 19th century the Army Medical Museum and Surgeon General's Office and Library joined. During the 20th century the organization was divided into different divisions. One became the leading pathological diagnostic laboratory and tumor registry in the world (The Armed Forces Institute of Pathology) and the historic material ultimately became the Otis Historical Archives of the National Museum of Health & Medicine. In 1986, historic medical photographs were returned from various governmental repositories and reorganized at the Otis Historical Archives.

THE DISCOVERY OF THE COLLECTION

My discovery and subsequent promotion of Bontecou and AMM medical photographs began in 1976, when I purchased a group of cartes de visite of Civil War wounded soldiers. Each was marked on the top of the photo with a number and "Contr. Photo." and some on the back were marked "AMM" with another number, and a card volume place identification. Others carried the stamped logo of a photographer: "R.B.B.- USV- Harewood." As one of the images was a tintype, a one of a kind photo, I realized that the group may be part of the original set that was contributed by physicians to the AMM during the Civil War. I contacted museum curators and began a three-decade search to uncover the story of the images and of "RBB."

In 1978, at Adelphi University's Swirbul Galleries, I exhibited my CdV images of Civil War wounded soldiers for the first time. Also in 1978, I began writing *Civil War Medical Photography*. It was published in 1980 and again in 1983 as part of my text, *Early Medical Photography in America (1839-1883)*. In this work I detailed the history of the use of photography by physicians in the Civil War and explained the nature of the clinical photographs. For completeness I surveyed all the known varieties of medical images taken in the war by, of, and for physicians. I reproduced pages from catalogues that listed the photographs that were in museum collections and also listed the texts in which the photographs were published as engravings. A history of not only clinical, but pathological and photomicrograph images, were presented along with the use of clinical images in the pension systems after the war. I clearly showed that most of the recognized Civil War clinical photographs were taken not during the war but after the war at the AMM for pension purposes and that for the most part only the images taken at Harewood, Lincoln and some other hospitals were original photographs produced during the war. *Civil War Medical Photography* remains to this day, perhaps the definitive review of the topic and is available from the Burns Archive. In 1979, (after *Civil War Medical Photography* went to the printer) I bought two albums originally owned by Bontecou. He had created these two albums from his CdV's collection with large format images with over 100 photographs in each album. The first volume showed healed wounds from head to hand, the second from upper body to foot. In some cases a CdV of the original injury or healed state was pasted on the back of the page with the larger photograph.

In the mid 1980s I bought another large format Bontecou album containing over 100 photographs. This was his personal teaching album and contained his signature in places and his hand drawings of the suspected paths of the wounding bullets. Images of wounded soldiers from other sources were loose in back of the album. As a coeditor of various medical journals I began to publish articles on Bontecou and his images. On June 22, 1986, I bought at auction from the estate of his granddaughter Marion Alice Bontecou the *Harewood Album: Wounded Soldiers*, containing 570 cartes de visite photographs. The album had been returned to the family in 1915 at the request of his son and is well documented by several letters. I was also able to buy some of his surgical instruments, personal photographs, office signs, images of his life in upstate New York, and images by his son Reed Brinsmade Bontecou, who was also a physician and served in the military in WWI. During the next year I interviewed and filmed his surviving

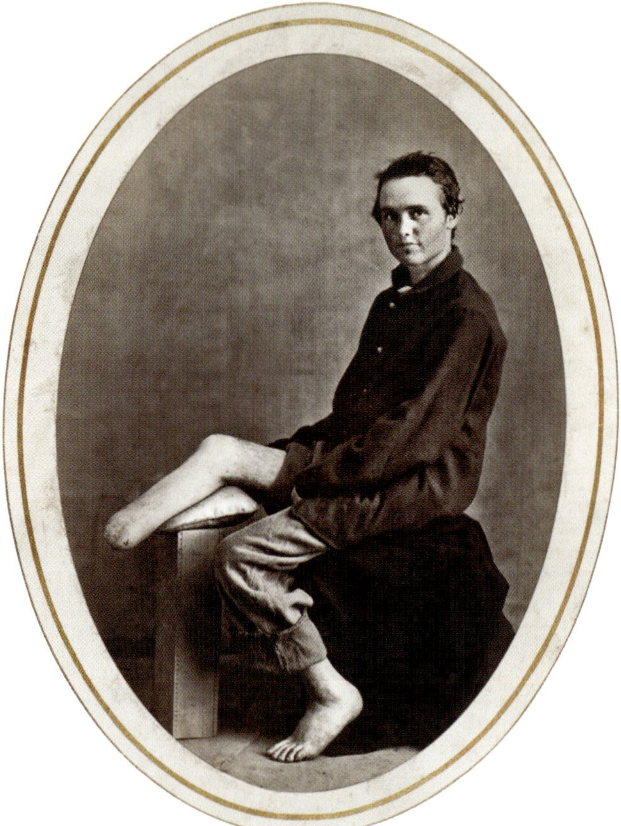

CHARLES FOX, PVT. CO. I 111 N.Y. VOLS. "AGED 18, ADMITTED APRIL 5TH, 1865 TO HAREWOOD HOSPITAL, SUFFERING FROM GSW RIGHT FOOT FRACTURING METATARSAL BONE OF BIG TOE AND SEVERELY INJURING OS CALCIS. WOUNDED MARCH 31ST, AT THE BATTLE OF PETERSBURGH, VA. ON ADMISSION, THE CONDITION OF INJURED PARTS, HOWEVER WAS TOLERABLE GOOD. PARTS BECAME SUBSEQUENTLY GANGRENOUS, WITH DISORGANIZATION OF THE ANKLE JOINT, BONES NECROSED AND SLOUGHING OF SOFT PARTS. SINUSES HAD FORMED, EXTENDED UPWARDS THE LEG. THE LIMB WAS AMPUTATED AT THE LOWER THIRD BY CIRCULAR METHOD. PATIENT DID WELL AFTER THE OPERATION UNDER SIMPLE DRESSING… PARTS NEARLY HEALED WHEN TRANSFERRED TO LINCOLN USA HOSPITAL JULY 20TH, 1865." PHOTOGRAPH FROM BONTECOU'S 5 1/2 BY 71/2 INCH TWO VOLUME SET OF BODY WOUNDS.

relatives including his grandchildren. They provided a direct emotional link to his life and his work. In November 1986 I published in *MD magazine* "A Doctors Civil War," detailing the significance of the discovery of the CdV album. In 1987, artist Joel-Peter Witkin, fascinated with deformity and wounds, requested to visit the AMM and review their clinical images of the Civil War. He was told by the curator, "the original images are in the Burns Collection." After several visits and survey of my collection he edited *Masterpieces of Medical Photography: Selections from the Burns Archive.* Dr. Bontecou's images dominated the book and were the core of an exhibit that traveled to several countries, firmly establishing Bontecou's place as a noted clinical and art photographer.

In 1990 four pages from the CdV album were published in Ken Burns' *The Civil War* and a few images were presented in his documentary of the same name. In 1992, at the request of curators at the Metropolitan Museum of Art (MMA), I donated seventeen of the photographs from Bontecou's personal 5 ½ by 7 ½ inch print teaching album. Several were put on exhibition at the museum. These images, supplemented with others from my collection, may form the core of a future exhibit at the museum. They can be seen on the MMA website. In 1993, Random House published *Face of Mercy: A Photographic History of Medicine at War*, I was the photo historian for the book supplying images and captions. In the chapter on the Civil War Bontecou's images were central to the story. By the mid-1990s other historians began to study his images and I supported their work by supplying imagery for their publications. During the 1990s, plastic surgeon Blair O. Rogers and I worked on various aspects of plastic surgery in war photography. In 1995 and 2000 he published articles on Bontecou's work in the field. In 1998, using some of Dr. Bontecou's CdV images, Jack Woody published *A Mornings Work: Medical Photographs from the Burns Collection & Archive (1839-1943).* The title came from Bontecou's caption for his photograph of a pile of amputated legs. This was the first time the famous image was seen in its original version. Previously I had published the cropped version that he made for his large print album. In 2003 I began publishing my medical specialty series. In each one Bontecou's photographs have highlighted medical and surgical conditions and represented the earliest known photograph of the disease or wound. In Spring 2011 in conjunction with the release of this text an exhibition of Bontecou photographs of New York wounded soldiers will be presented at New York City's Merchant House Museum. Other venues will include The National Museum of Civil War Medicine as the Bontecou series is published during the Sesquicentennial.

THE SPECIMEN COLLECTOR

I have copies of most of Bontecou's correspondence with military authorities. Bontecou was proud of his wartime achievement and in his later years proudly noted: "The index of the Surgical History of the War gives me credit as its largest contributor and I was the first to apply Photography to the Military history of the soldier while I was in charge of Harewood, U.S.A. Gen'l Hospital at Washington, D.C. in 1864."

Ever since the 1840s, when he collected specimens in the Amazon for a Troy, NY museum, Bontecou had a penchant for collecting objects for study and began acquiring war medical specimens before the government's proclamations. Collecting body parts for study was a time honored medical tradition and noted doctors had their own museums. Bontecou's first major donation to the AMM was in May 1863 with specimens from Hygeia Hospital. He lists "88 morbid (pathological) specimens categories" (heads, arms. legs, bones, projectiles, etc.) from General McClellan's 1862 ill-fated peninsular campaign. In a letter dated Feb. 10, 1863 Surgeon General Hammond accuses him of having about 300 specimens which rightfully belonged to the AMM. Bontecou responded that about 30 anatomical wet preparations "were accidentally destroyed by negroes who cleaned the dead house," and others were given to physicians. He reported he would work to retrieve the specimens for the AMM as they were given away before official orders to collect specimens for a museum were received. The human heads Bontecou harvested were unidentified but he recorded "heads of rebels" from Alabama, Mississippi, South Carolina, and one of a negro rebel sharpshooter. Bontecou asked Dr. Hammond to let him keep some of the heads that did not have gun shot wounds. The study of heads and skulls in this time was an important part of psychiatry, neurology and physical anthropology. It was believed that behavioral, racial, and criminal attitudes could be identified by measuring and studying heads. One of the government's first official research projects was in skull measurements. This also helps explain Bontecou's actions when visiting the Wilderness and Spotsylvania battlefields in March, 1866 he collected "Confederate" skulls for study and donated most of them to the AMM. In the chapter "Death and Sacrifice," I discuss the general disregard for identification and proper burial of servicemen. Confederate soldiers' bodies were treated with little respect and were often simply left to rot. On Oct. 27, 1873 he sent "two boxes containing thirty skulls & severed bone specimens exhibiting gunshot injuries." The museum still has this collection. Bontecou apparently thrived in his work at Harewood. After arriving home in Troy, NY Bontecou writes Surgeon General Otis: "I look back at my life in Washington with regrets that it could not last always."

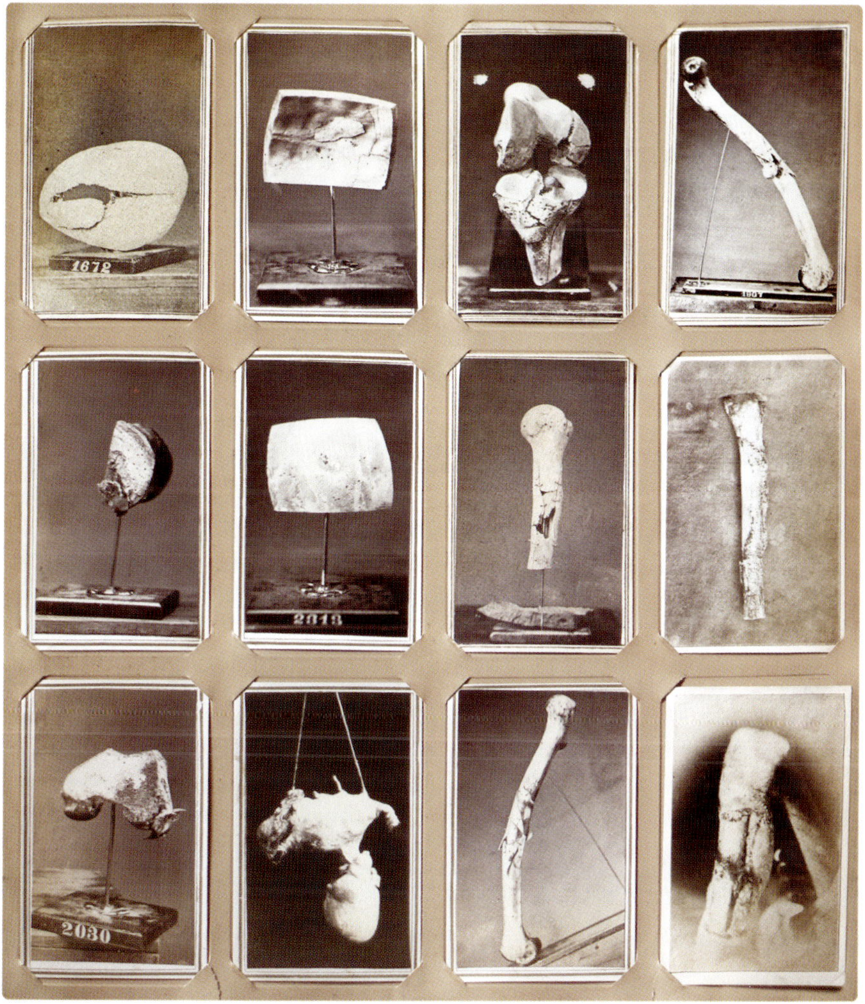

BONTECOU PHOTOGRAPHED THE BONE SPECIMEN HE DONATED TO THE ARMY MEDICAL MUSEUM AND PLACED SOME OF THE IMAGES IN HIS CDV ALBUM.

REED BROCKWAY BONTECOU, MD: A SURGEON'S LIFE

Reed Bontecou was born in Troy, New York on April 22, 1824. His parents were of Huguenot and Scottish descent. He was a descendent of David Bontecou one of the original Huguenot settlers of Connecticut. The Bontecou clan, according to two texts from the 1880s, are descended from early European nobility. The founder of the family was Pipin the Old, born in 560. His great-great-grandson was Charles Martel who defeated the Moslem Armies at the Battle of Tours in 752, freeing Europe from Mohammedan influence. Pepin the Short born 715, and Charlemagne, born 742, Emperor of the West were other predecessors, hence the family's claim to their short stature. Bontecou physicians had lived in Holland and were trained at the University of Leiden. Among Bontecou's fore bearers was noted seamen among them Willem Ysbrandtsz Bontekoe (1587-1657) the captain of a Dutch ship the Bontekoe, his 1646 published journal on his 1618 voyage for the Dutch East India Company made him famous and in 2007 a film was made on one aspect of his journal. In 1660 a ship named De Bontekoe sailed from Holland to New York bringing cargo and immigrants.

Dr. Bontecou was educated in Troy. After graduating from Troy High School he went to the Rensselaer Polytechnic Institute from which he graduated in 1842. Here his love for the natural sciences was stimulated and inspired by Professor Amos Eaton and Bontecou became a serious ornithologist. About this time two Troy physicians convinced him to study medicine and he entered the offices of Drs. Wright, Skilton and Brinsmade with the three physicians as preceptors for his medical training. He spent almost two years in this preceptorship then for about two years, 1844-1845, he attended lectures in the medical department of the recently founded University of the City of New York. Dr Skilton was also a natural scientist of note and he and Bontecou spent a good deal of time differentiating and classifying seashells. In 1846, with his natural science interest rekindled, he took a break from his medical studies. He went to South America to help the Troy Elysium of Natural History to collect specimens. He spent the entire year collecting flora and fauna along the Amazon River and brought back hundreds of birds and other specimens. In later years Dr. Bontecou would decorate his office with these bird specimens, which his children and grandchildren fondly remembered.

When he returned to Troy he learned of the death of his friend and preceptor, Dr. John Wright and on the advice of Dr. Thomas Brinsmade, Bontecou enrolled in Castleton Vermont Medical College to officially obtain his medical degree. After graduation in

May 1847, he formed a partnership with Dr. Brinsmade. It was a special partnership, while both doctors saw general patients; Bontecou would do all the surgical work. In 1849 he married a cousin, Susanna Bontecou Northrup. They had five children; Joanna, b. 1850-d.1852; Anna Louise b.1851-d.1872; Josephine b.1856-d.1911; Horatio b.1861-d. 1862, and Reed Brinsmade Bontecou, Dec 1, 1864- Jun 18,1943, who became a physician and continued his father's practice in Troy. Bontecou practiced medicine for the next 56 years, retiring in 1903. He was an indefatigable worker and had a skill "not exceeded by many other American surgeons." His manual dexterity and skillful manner with which he handled the knife along with his quick operating time, resulted in lessened shock and greater surgical success. Because of his short stature he was known as the "Little Napoleon with a Scalpel." Bontecou's pre-war experiences and attitude ultimately made him perhaps the most successful general hospital surgeon of the Civil War.

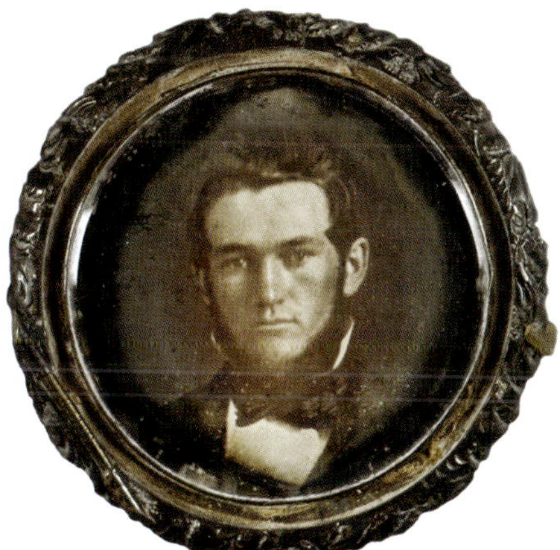

DR. BONTECOU, DAGUERREOTYPE LOCKET, CIRCA 1855.

EARLY CAREER

In 1848 Bontecou went to New York City to study cholera, to learn its clinical features and the therapeutic measures available at the time. By the time he returned to Troy, cholera had struck and continued to strike the city until 1855. Bontecou was in charge of the Troy hospital in 1857 when cholera struck yet again. Among the constant terrors of the time was diphtheria, which he treated by placing patients in large well-ventilated rooms with open windows, even in winter. When airway obstruction was threatened he performed tracheotomy. Aside from routine surgery Bontecou reported several unusual surgical and medical cases. He was one of the pioneers of opium therapy in peritonitis, using it since 1848. One of his early important therapeutic triumphs occurred in 1854 when he successfully used opium to treat general peritonitis. His most famous and fascinating case occurred in August 1854: "Mrs. W.A. a 34 year old, six months pregnant woman while in a squatting position feeding her chickens ruptured an old umbilical hernia of large dimension. Nearly all of her intestines fell to the dirty ground." Bontecou was the last of several physicians who saw her. The previous ones stated nothing could be done and left her to her fate. This do-nothing-attitude for abdominal wounds was the general practice of the time as peritonitis killed the patient in a few days. It was a lingering, painful death, and so much more so for a pregnant woman whose intestines fell on chicken stool infected dirt. By the time Bontecou saw her late that night, the patient was in shock and her exposed viscera was covered with dirt and swollen to immense size. In spite of the seeming hopelessness of the situation, Bontecou went into action: he cleaned her intestines, surgically enlarged the wound in her abdomen and managed, after much effort, to replace the swollen intestines. He then took the edges of the skin of the torn hernial sack and closed it with large hatpins. He applied a bandage and gave her a dose of morphine large enough to let her die easily. Surprisingly the patient was alive next day, in spite of severe peritonitis. Bontecou continued to administer repeated large doses of opium (15-20 grains). Miraculously the patient recovered and about a month after had a premature delivery. She subsequently had several other children. During the war, this experience made Bontecou an advocate of aggressively treating abdominal wounds, even those with peritonitis.

In the 19th century cervical fractures were usually fatal. On April 3, 1856, a man suffered a fracture of the cervical vertebrae with complete paralysis of motion and sensation in the trunk and all four extremities. Bontecou treated him successfully by pulley extension and counter extension with use of plaster of Paris casts. In a few months the patient's fracture healed and he recovered sufficiently to pursue his occupation as a house painter. When the patient died from liver disease 20 years later, an autopsy by Bontecou verified the diagnosis of the fracture. In 1857 Dr. Bontecou performed the first case in

North America where the subclavian artery was tied for a diffuse traumatic aneurysm, it was one of the first three successful cases on record. The patient had dislocated his right shoulder with a resultant traumatic aneurysm of the axillary artery. The operation took one hour on Nov. 21, 1857. He published the case in the *Transactions of the Medical Society of New York* in 1858.

MILITARY CAREER

Aside from all his medical and surgical war accomplishments Bontecou had the distinction of being a surgeon in the first volunteer Union regiment of the Civil War. He did his first work in the first official battle of the war and he was perhaps the last volunteer surgeon to be discharged (June 6, 1866).

Bontecou's military experience began more than a decade before the war. On August 5, 1849 New York State Governor Edwin Morgan commissioned him a surgeon of the 24th Regiment, 10th Brigade, 3rd Division of the New York State Militia. He served in that capacity for the next decade. When the Civil War started Bontecou was one of the first to answer the call of his country. He joined the regiment on April 24, 1861 and was mustered into US service on May 14, 1861. He was commissioned as surgeon of the 2nd NY Infantry (First Troy Regiment), one of the first volunteer regiments of Union soldiers. While surgeon to this regiment he performed his first operations on the field at the Battle of Big Bethel, the first battle of the war. This battle was fought on June 10th, 1861, less than a month after his appointment and 31 days before the famous Battle at Bull Run. Big Bethel Virginia is just north of Fort Monroe. Generals Benjamin Butler and Ebenezer Pierce led 4,400 Federal troops, mostly New York regiments, against 1,400 entrenched Confederates. It was a Confederate victory and as one union officer commented a "Federal disaster." The battle truly forecast future events. Only one rebel was killed and 7 wounded while the Union had 18 killed and 53 wounded. (Henry Lawson Wyatt Co G 1st North Carolina is memorialized as the first CSA soldier killed in the war). It was also at this battle that uniform color was established. Federal troops had fired on Federal troops! The 7th New York fired on the 3rd New York, as the 3rd were dressed in grey uniforms and were located behind the 7th. When the 7th thought they were being surrounded, they killed 2 and wounded 21. Blue would become the standard

Federal issue uniform. Dr Bontecou's penchant for souvenirs and recording events is evident by his bloodstained wallet that survives from Big Bethel, in it three coins and a note: "These coins were driven into a soldier's groin by a bullet in the War of the Rebellion."

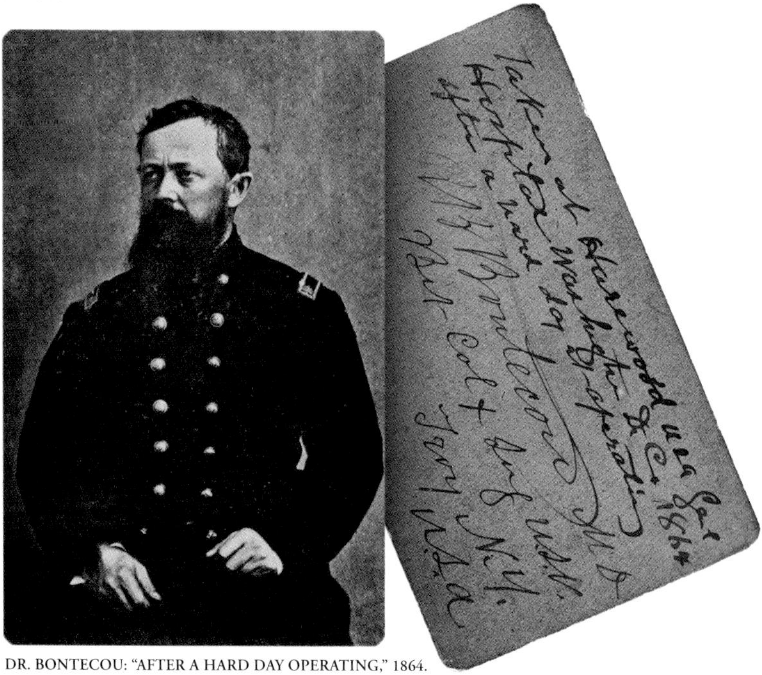

DR. BONTECOU: "AFTER A HARD DAY OPERATING," 1864.

Because of Bontecou's outstanding performance at Big Bethel, he was examined by a special board in Washington, DC and on September 14th, 1861 was promoted to Brigade Surgeon US Volunteers and placed in charge of the Hygeia US Army General Hospital at Fortress Monroe, Virginia. While at Hygeia Hospital in the winter of 1861 Bontecou performed the first resection of a shoulder joint reported to the surgeon general's office. The result was a success and the arm was restored to usefulness. The innovation paved the way for new aggressive surgical therapy.

Records at the National Archive note: "To quarantine patients, Bontecou established a small pox hospital on the beach a mile north of the main hospital at the fort. Bontecou was obliged to inspect the small pox disease. While returning from such duty on the evening of February 25, 1862, Bontecou ran his horse along the beach. In the dark his horse tripped over the partly-buried carcass of a mule & fell, throwing him violently over its head and causing a hernia at the umbilicus. The injury was not permanently disabling, but nonetheless the Doctor was confined to his room... 'Twas several days before he was able to resume his duties. On Sunday morning, March 9, 1862, Bontecou [still suffering from his injury] was assisted to the lookout on the roof of the Hygeia Hospital." There he watched the historic engagement between the *Monitor* and *Virginia* on the waters of Hampton Roads.

Fortress Monroe and Hygeia Hospital are at the end of a peninsula that extends out into Hampton Roads, which is the name of the waterway to the bay outlet of the James River. As Federal ships blockaded the bay the Confederate navy attempted to break through with a new weapon of war: the ironclad battleship. As a consequence of Fort Monroe's position, Bontecou observed and may have assisted at the world famous first battle of ironclad warships—the USS *Monitor* (built in his home town of Troy) and the *CSS Virginia* also known as the *Merrimac*. Known as the Battle of Hampton Roads it was fought over two days, March 8th and 9th, 1862. Bontecou was stationed with signalmen as a lookout on the roof of Hygeia Hospital during the battle, it was one of the closest pieces of land to the entire battle and was near the entrance to the harbor. On March 9, after trading hundreds of rounds of cannon fire, the battle was a stalemate but it ushered in a new era in naval warfare. Soon after the naval battle Federal General George McClellan began his ill-fated Peninsular Campaign. As a result of the exposed position of Hygeia Hospital on the peninsular, Bontecou was ordered to close the hospital on August 30th. It was destroyed by Confederate forces on September 2nd. Bontecou was then detailed to the Army of the Potomac and served as a surgeon in the Second Battle of Bull Run. At this time he was in the Office of the Surgeon General in Washington DC making many influential friends. But he had caught malaria. After receiving orders to report to Hilton Head South Carolina, in a letter dated September 12th 1862 to Surgeon General Hammond, Bontecou writes, "Permit me respectfully to ask for duty somewhere north of the Potomac. I have not yet fully recovered from the effects of fever I suffered during the month of August at Fort Monroe and am apprehensive that removal to a hot climate

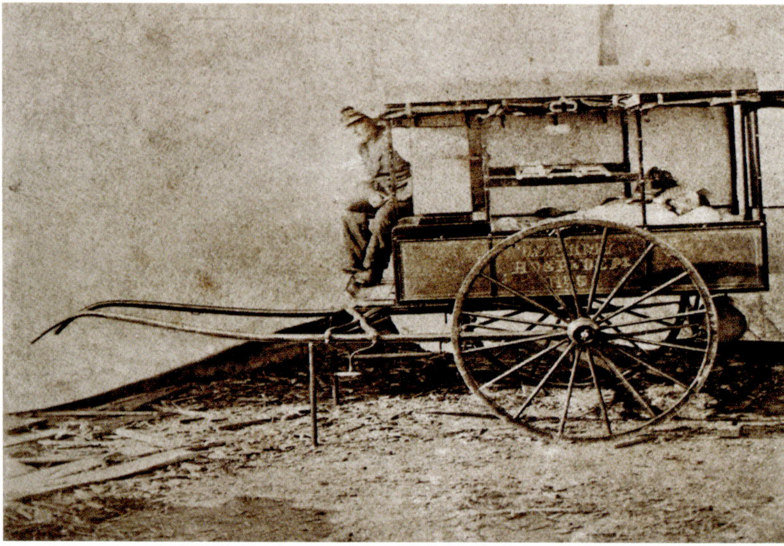

DREADED TWO WHEELED AMBULANCES AGGRAVATED WOUNDS BY THEIR ROUGH RIDE. RARE VIEW, ORIGINALLY IN THE ARMY MEDICAL MUSEUM COLLECTION, 1864.

at this time may render me unfit for service." After a short stay in New York City at the Astor Hotel Bontecou received his orders to South Carolina. There he supervised the US Army Hospital No. 1 in Beaufort beginning this assignment on October 1st. Soon after arriving at Beaufort he attended Union General Ormsby M. Mitchell, Commander of the Department of the South, who was dying of yellow fever. He died Oct 30. Mitchell is best remembered as a staunch opponent of the "soft war" and for his support of slave rights and confiscating Confederate properties for the benefit of slaves. Bontecou was soon appointed chief medical officer supervising the ten South Carolina general military hospitals. While in South Carolina he served with his friend Assistant Surgeon General Charles Crane on the USS *Monitor* during the futile attack on Confederate held Fort Sumter in Charleston Harbor.

On April 7, 1863 nine iron clad Union ships, seven new Passaic class versions of the *USS Monitor*, the experimental iron clad *USS Keokuk* along with the *USS Monitor* attacked Ft. Sumter in Charleston Harbor. Bontecou was on board the *USS Monitor* with Assistant Surgeon General Crane as combat surgeons. The attack failed, as did the

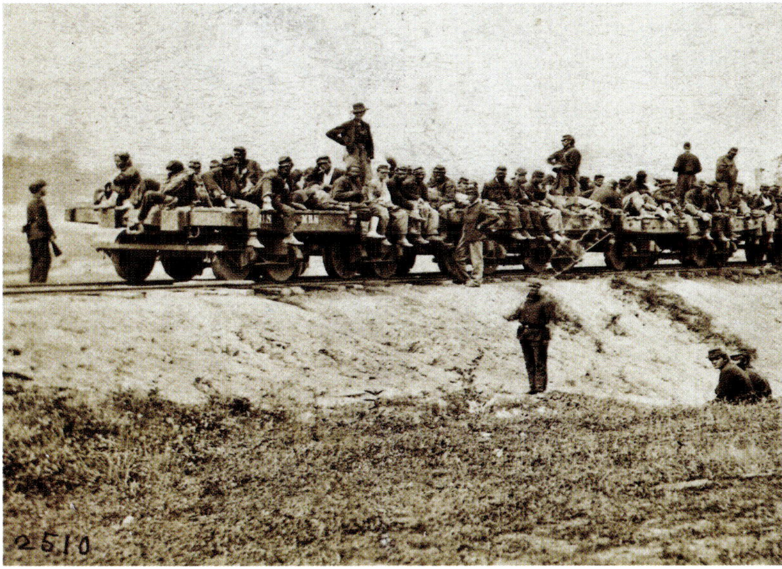

FLAT CARS LOADED WITH WOUNDED SOLDIERS, McCLELLAN'S PENINSULA CAMPAIGN, JUNE 1862.

Second Battle of Sumter on September 1-2, 1863. On April 25, 1863 he wrote the army commander at Hilton Head: "I have respectfully to request a leave of absence for ten days to go to New York City on account of affliction in my family having lost by death one of my children (Horatio) in the present week." He returned to Hilton Head in early May. On May 24, 1863 Bontecou was placed in charge of the large hospital ship *Cosmopolitan*, which lay off Charleston. His job was to convey the sick and wounded from various points on the Atlantic coast to large general hospitals from Key West to New York City. This service in South Carolina put him in place to participate in one of the great episodes of the war. I have nicknamed Bontecou "Surgeon of Glory" for he was the surgeon in charge of taking care of the African American soldiers of the famed Massachusetts 54th and 55th Colored Troop regiments, wounded at the ill fated battle for Fort Wagner on Morris Island as depicted in the movie *Glory*. While Bontecou himself did not write a report on this episode in the M*edical and Surgical History of the War of the Rebellion,* Vol. 1 of Part 1-*Medical History* p.242, Dr. J.J. Craven tells of Bontecou's role in the two fruitless Battles for Fort Wagner on Morris Island, July 11 and July 18, 1863.

EXTRACT FROM A REPORT ON WOUNDED AFTER THE ASSAULT ON FORT WAGNER IN JULY 1863 BY SURGEON J. J. CRAVEN, U.S. VOLUNTEERS

MEDICAL SURGICAL HISTORY OF THE WAR OF THE REBELLION, PART I - VOL I MEDICAL HISTORY P241 (B ON P242)

"On the morning of the 11th, an unsuccessful assault being made upon Fort Wagner, I commenced removing the wounded to the boats, and forwarding them to Folly Island. Learning that the hospital steamer Cosmopolitan *had reached Stono Inlet, and anchored at Pawnee Landing, on the opposite side of the island, less than half a mile from the beach hospital I dispatched a communication directing Surgeon Bontecou, U.S.V., in charge of the* Cosmopolitan *to commence the removal of the wounded from the beach to the* Cosmopolitan. * * *In the charge of the morning of the 11th, there were eleven killed, ninety-nine wounded, and one hundred missing."* (Bontecou removed the wounded and returned to the area. This was the first battle of Fort Wagner a week later the more famous battle occurred: Dr Craven continues:) *" On the night of the 18th, at dark, an attack was made upon Fort Wagner. At nine o'clock the firing ceased, and the ambulance train advanced to the front, near enemy lines, and commenced the transportation of the wounded. The killed, wounded and missing in this attack amounted to one thousand two hundred and sixty-eight.* * * *The island being exposed, and not knowing what advantage the enemy might take, while we were in a crippled condition, I thought it best to remove all the wounded from the island… sent a courier to the steamer* Cosmopolitan *with an order directing Surgeon R. B. Bontecou, U. S. V., to proceed with his hospital ship to the mouth of the Stono, and in smooth water just inside of the bar, anchor and await the coming of the Alice Price, upon which steamer I immediately place two hundred and forty wounded men and she proceeded to Stono, where her load was transferred to the* Cosmopolitan i*n two hours. The Alice Price was under the charge of Surgeon A.C. Barlow, 62nd Ohio Volunteers and Surgeon Stone 54th Massachusetts Volunteers. Knowing that the* Cosmopolitan *had as many as she could accommodate, I directed Surgeon Bontecou to proceed to Hilton Head immediately…. By the direction of General Gilmore, I proceeded to the front, and under a flag of truce, communicated with General Hagood of the Confederate army, commandant of Fort Wagner, with whom we negotiated for an exchange of wounded, naming the following Friday morning at ten o'clock, as the time when I would meet a Confederate steamer in Charleston harbor.*

I returned to Hilton Head, and placed all the rebel wounded upon the Cosmopolitan, *whence I returned to Charleston harbor meeting the Confederate steamer Alice, and delivered to the officers in charge of the flag, thirty-nine wounded Confederates. * * We received on board the* Cosmopolitan, *from the officers in charge of the Alice, one hundred and five wounded officers and men. The officers in charge of the Alice reported still remaining in hospitals at Charleston one hundred and eight officers and men, and dead in their hands fifty-one. * * As soon as the transfer was made, the* Cosmopolitan *conveyed our wounded to Hilton Head."*

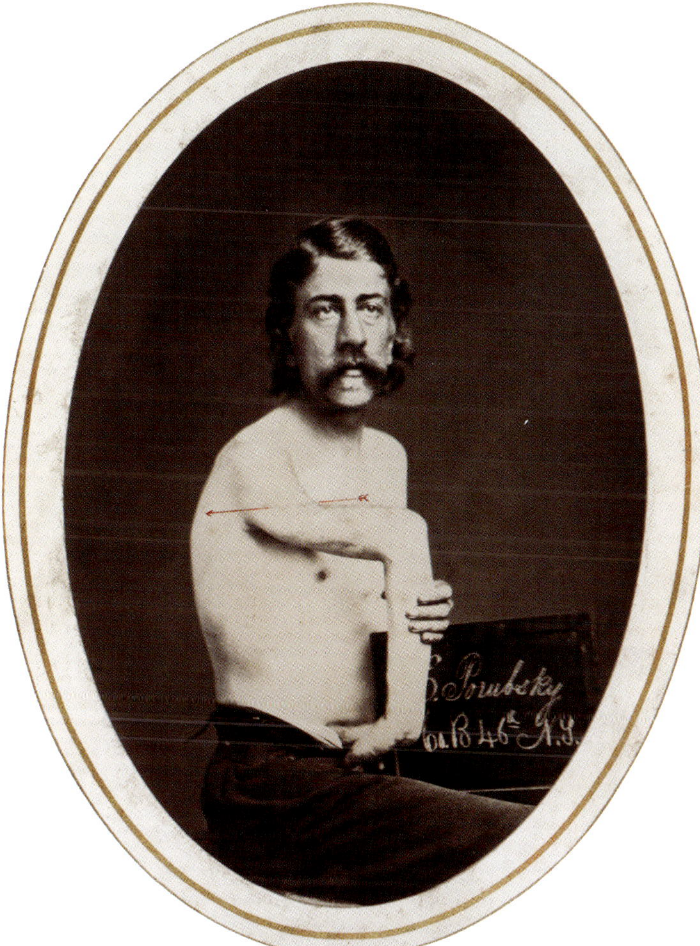

G. PORUBSKY, CO B. 46TH NY VOLUNTEER DISPLAYING EXCISION OF HUMERUS. THIS PHOTOGRAPH FROM BONTECOU'S TEACHING ALBUM SHOWS THE DRAWN-IN SUSPECTED PATH OF THE BULLET. BONTECOU'S OPERATION OF BONE REMOVAL IN THE UPPER ARM LEFT THE PATIENT WITH A USELESS LIMB. MANY WERE AMPUTATED IN THE ANTISEPTIC SURGICAL ERA OF THE 1880s.

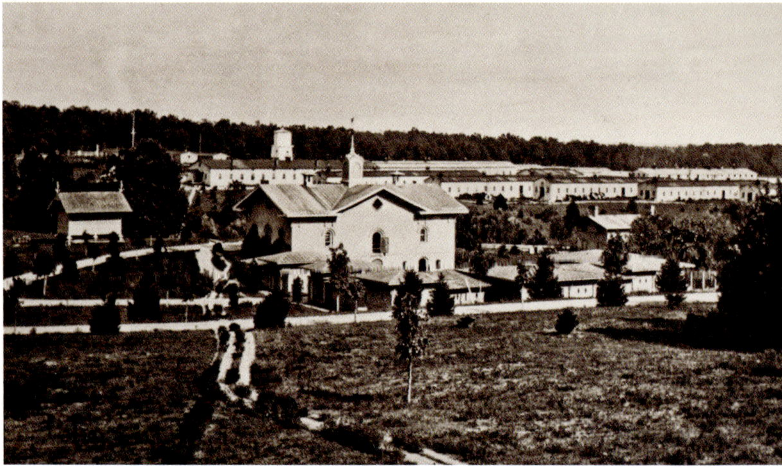

HAREWOOD US ARMY GENERAL HOSPITAL WASHINGTON D.C.

Bontecou's previous friendships and duties with Assistant Surgeon General Crane and others in Washington, combined with his outstanding performance in the field, resulted in his appointment in October 1863 to assume charge of Harewood United States Army General Hospital, with its three thousand beds on three hundred acres in the suburbs of Washington DC. By the end of the war Harewood was perhaps the largest functioning Union hospital.

It was at Harewood that Bontecou introduced the application of photography for clinical purposes. He remained in charge of the hospital, with its enormous medical and surgical services, until June 6, 1866. Bontecou had gained fame as a surgeon for practicing excisions and resections of gunshot injuries to bones in the extremities, instead of performing amputations. He photographed the results of these operations. Unfortunately time would show that this practice of excising shattered bones in the upper extremity, done so that the limb did not have to be amputated, turned out not to be the best therapy since a boneless arm was almost useless. In the antiseptic surgical era established in the 1880s many of the limbs 'without long bones' were amputated.

At Harewood Hospital, Bontecou performed the first resection of a knee joint to treat a gunshot injury. He photographed this operation and the images are in the CdV album. He also devised a conservative operation on the foot, modifying the famed Russian surgeon Pirigoff's operation so that it could be performed with more ease. Bontecou's personality, social contacts and beliefs are gradually being uncovered and indications as to his character are unfolding. One episode at Harewood seems quite interesting as he almost lost his military career over it. On December 15, 1863, Captain R. L. Ayers wrote the commander of the 9th USA Regiment, Col. George W. Giles, concerning Bontecou's aberrant actions. He reported that Bontecou befriended a rebel prisoner and patient at the hospital, John A. Adams of the Louisiana Guard Artillery, "who was only slightly wounded by a blow to the head and should have been sent to the Old Capitol Prison in early November." Bontecou had invited Adams to Thanksgiving dinner at his home on November 26, 1863 and also to lunch on December 13th. Adams bragged about his favorable treatment to other patients. Eleven personnel, including nine assistant surgeons, were listed as providing evidence of the events. On Jan 4th Col. Hoffman, of the 3rd Infantry, after documenting Ayer's letter, writes to the Office of General of Prisoners: "For this neglect the surgeon in whose immediate charge and the surgeon in charge of the hospital, are equally responsible…visiting Surgeon Bontecou…which, if not in violation of his orders, was a plain violation of propriety in such cases. For these neglects of his duty I would respectfully suggest that Surgeon Bontecou be removed from the charge of the Harewood Hospital." On Jan 7th the matter was referred to the Surgeon General's Office and on Jan 9th Acting Surgeon General Joseph Barnes wrote, "as a result of Surgeon Bontecou's arduous duty, distinguished career, professional skill and zealous discharge of all his duties and the probability that no repetition of the incident will occur, no action will be taken against him." Bontecou continued as surgeon in charge until mid 1866. In the last months of his service he was on special boards related to artificial limb devices.

Bontecou introduced the concept of photographing soldiers' original wounds and the post-operative healed state. The images became a major educational device to help surgeons learn routine procedures and the expected results. He photographed not only all his interesting cases but took photographs of actual operative details, the first pictures of their kind ever taken anywhere. As the CdVs were probably taken with a four-lens camera, Bontecou contributed copies of many of his photographs to the Army Medical Museum and these images became the museum's central core of medical photographs.

In the noteworthy *Medical and Surgical History of the War of the Rebellion*, Bontecou is credited with being the largest contributor to the publication. He is also credited as the largest contributor of photographs to the Army Medical Museum, to which he also donated hundreds of specimens of bones and projectiles. The publications of the Surgeon General's Office are liberally illustrated with engravings from photographs of Bontecou's most interesting cases, some of which are published as photographs in this volume for the first time.

POST WAR CAREER

When the war ended in April 1865, Harewood Hospital was filled to capacity for several months. Bontecou stayed on as its chief, operating and treating those from the final assaults of the Petersburg and Appomattox campaigns. Sick and wounded patients lingered for months until they healed or died from infections. On June 15th, 1865 he was promoted to the rank of Lieutenant Colonel of Volunteers by brevet. The honor was bestowed as a result of meritorious service in the war. Harewood remained open at the war's end and received soldiers from other hospitals as they closed. When work slowed down in the spring of 1866, Bontecou asked for and received permission to tour the battlefields of the Wilderness and Spotsylvania. Between April 6th and the 14th Bontecou teamed with photographer William Bell, who was then working part time for the army, and together they made photographs of the battle grounds which, unfortunately, have been lost. Harewood was the last of the large general hospitals to close and Bontecou was among the last of the volunteer surgeons mustered out of service. In June 1866 Bontecou requested 20 days leave for important personal business in Troy. Instead of leave, he was mustered out of the service as the war had been over for fourteen months. On June 22, 1867 General Order No. 65 was issued, which promoted Bontecou to the rank of Colonel of Volunteers, by brevet, "to be dated from March 13, 1865."

Soon after his discharge he was offered the professorship of surgery at the distinguished St. Louis Medical College. He declined, preferring to remain in the town of his birth. He moved back to Troy and lived at 82 Fourth Street practicing general medicine and surgery. On January 1, 1872 Bontecou came under contract with the Watervliet Arsenal in West Troy NY at a salary of $50.00 per month. He was appointed Acting Assistant Surgeon, US Army at the arsenal. He examined recruits and especially Civil War pensioners, many of them wounded soldiers he had treated and had operated on during the war. One important task of post war physicians was performing pension examinations and certifying war related injuries and disease as veterans sought disability claims. A primary use of the CdV photographs was as proof of war injury or disease and they were often attached to soldiers pension records. These are now housed at the National Archives. In 1873 Bontecou's salary was raised to $100.00 per month and he continued to work at the arsenal into the 1890s.

In his practice Bontecou continued to perfect and pioneer surgical procedures. Back in 1858, while treating his friend Professor W. P. Seymour, with what would soon be recognized as appendicitis, the doctors discussed the condition and noted that the best way to treat the disease was to cut down to the abscess before peritonitis set in. They did not report their theory, however, and it was not until 1869 that Bontecou operated upon a case of appendicitis. This was one year after Dr. Willard Parker performed the first successful operation. In 1873 Bontecou reported three cases of appendicular abscess and curtenities (cicatricial) release by operation. He routinely ligated aneurisms and performed numerous ovariectomies, hysterectomies, lithotomies and procedures for strangulated hernia, all with great success. In 1897 he made the first attempt in the United States, and the second in the world by any surgeon, to repair a typhoidal intestinal perforation. The operation, however, was unsuccessful.

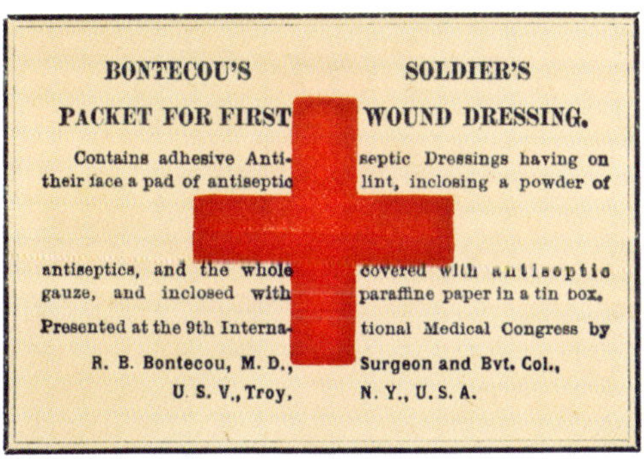

With the introduction of aseptic wound considerations in the mid 1880s Bontecou created the first antiseptic wound packet that could be used by an individual soldier. His unique portable kit would allow each soldier to antiseptically dress his own wound until professional aid arrived. In September 1887, he read two papers at at the Section of at the Ninth International Medical Congress, Washington, D.C.: "What Class of Gunshot Wounds and Injuries Justify Resection or Excision in Modern Warfare" along with "A Description of an Antiseptic Provisional Wound Dressing for the Field: Devised for the Military Service." Military authorities recognized the need for the field dressing but thought it should only be issued to a few designated servicemen (corpsmen) as it would be too costly to give every serviceman a kit since not all servicemen were wounded. By World War II every serviceman had a first aid pack. Today, in conflicts where improvised explosive devices (IEDs, most commonly roadside bombs) are used, some servicemen wear loose tourniquets around each arm and leg so that when wounded they can tighten the device and save their own lives, as blood loss is the leading cause of death.

Bontecou liked teaching and would send his students around to his patients' homes to record cases and make their own individual judgments. He received numerous honors during his final years. He was a popular teacher and an active member of the Rensselear Medical Society. He was its president in 1891 and 1892. On November 18, 1903 the Rensselear County Medical Society honored Bontecou at a special dinner. He was presented with a silver cup for his contributions to medicine and a photograph was made at the occasion (see title page). Bontecou died on March 7, 1907 and is buried in Oakwood Cemetery in Troy, New York. Bontecou's son Reed Brinsmade Bontecou (named after his medical partner) followed in his father's footsteps and served as a military surgeon in World War I. He was a member of the Troy National Guard Co A, 2nd Regiment. Both Dr. Bontecou's were avid photographers, as packets of film boxes with family photographs indicate.

While Bontecou's professional life was exemplary, his home life was not as peaceful or ideal. The November 29th 1883 *New York Times* reported that Susan Bontecou was granted a divorce from Reed who was "alleged to have criminal intimacy with Emma Josephine Murray, known as Emma Brockway. The court granted Susan $200 counsel fees and $1,750 per year for maintenance of herself and the two children. The testimony was not made public. The parties all move in the highest social circles of this city (Troy)." Susan and her daughter Josephine moved to Europe for adventure and to start new lives, Susan to see the classic scenes of Europe, Josephine to study medicine, psychology and write fiction. They lived in Leipzig Germany. Bontecou's daughter would achieve some notoriety in her own right. At a lecture by Wilhelm Wundt, the pioneer experimental psychologist, she met a man ten years her junior, Lincoln Steffens (1866-1936). He was to become a noted American investigative journalist and muckraker. Josephine was headed to Paris to study anatomy at the Sorbonne and psychology with neuropsychiatrist Jean-Martin Charcot. Steffens followed and their romance blossomed as they committed to an unconventional relationship. In 1891 they married in Paris. Susan Bontecou supported them until the couple returned to America in 1892, as Steffans had landed a job at the

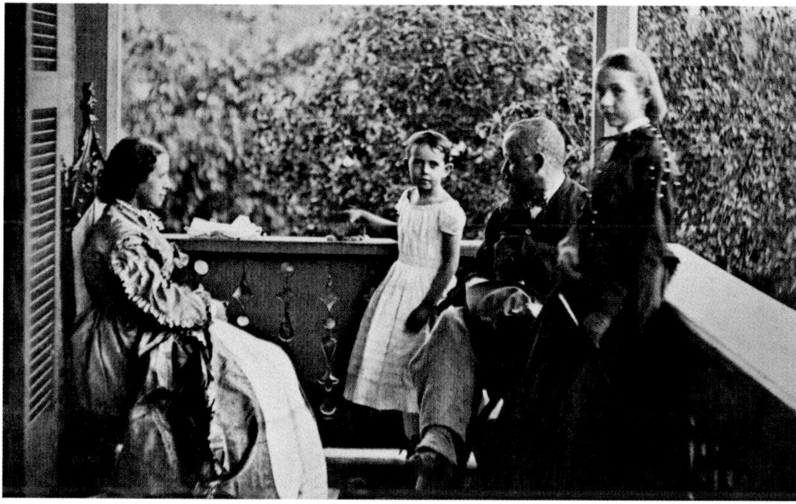

THE BONTECOU FAMILY ON THE FRONT PORCH OF THEIR HOME IN WASHINGTON, DC, 1864. SUSAN (PREGNANT WITH REED JR.), ANITA LOUISE (WHITE DRESS), JOSEPHINE ON BONTECOU'S LEFT.

New York Evening Post. Later he became editor of *McClure's Magazine.* He hounded corrupt city officials across America with his exposés of wrongdoing and was responsible for dozens to be ousted, indicted or jailed. His 1904 book *Shame of the Cities* was a best seller. Josephine became a novelist and in 1899 published *Letitia Berkley.* She was also known for her support of open unconventional relationships. Josephine died in 1911. They had no children.

In the summer of 1986 I was invited to a family gathering where I interviewed the Bontecou clan. A few of Bontecou's grandchildren were still alive. The family generously supplemented the album with numerous personal photographs of Bontecou during the war and subsequent years. His grandchildren remembered personal stories about him and they provided a personality profile of their illustrious granddad. One family tale purported that Reed Bontecou Sr. was a grave robber and leader of a group that got thrown out of Troy because he was trying to dry cadaver bones on the roof of his house. None of his grandchildren became physicians. His granddaughter Marion, who had the album and recently died, had a phobia and no one could touch anything in the house, including the cartes de visite album.

THE NEW DEADLY WEAPON

Every war has a game-changing weapon. The new weapon's effect is usually not appreciated by old-line professional soldiers who continue to use the last war's tactics, often to the detriment of the frontline servicemen. The improvised explosive device (IED) is today's new horror weapon and in the Civil War the Minie Ball, a bullet–shaped (conical-cylindrical shape) soft lead bullet invented by Claude Etienne Minié, was the new weapon. It made the close-line formations of soldiers shooting at each other from a few yards away obsolete, yet almost all battles of the Civil War were fought in that style. Muskets used round lead balls. These round balls, rammed down a muzzle loading weapon, did not fit tightly and as a result were not accurate and did not have the penetrating power of the new 58 caliber Minie Ball. These new projectiles had grooves and an iron core that expanded the lead and locked it tightly into the rifle barrel for greater accuracy and power. It was a spin-stabilized projectile. The Minie Ball, like the old round lead ball, shattered and fractured bone easily and commonly carried clothing and other debris with it into the wound, making infection a constant companion in almost every case. Soldiers of the time spread rumors about the power of the projectile; that at over 1,200 yards (about 2/3 of a mile) the bullet could penetrate a soldier and his knapsack and still kill anyone standing behind him and at very close distances could kill every person in a line of 15. In May 1864 at Spotsylvania, John Sedgwick, the highest ranking Union general killed in the war, was shot by a sniper in the face at 800 yards as he chided his men about their being afraid of rebel sharpshooters. In reality the regular issue military weapons using Minie Balls were accurate to at least 300 yards compared to the round musket ball at only 100 yards. By 1863 some troops were issued breech loading and multi shot weapons. Over 94% of Federal wounds were caused by bullet, 5.5% by artillery and less than 0.4% by bayonet or saber.

The wounding of bodies is one of the important goals of war. The new bullets certainly helped with this goal. A dead body requires no assistance but a wounded body requires assistance, care, and treatment, even after the war. The wounded provide a populace with constant reminders of the human cost of war. The dead are a statistic but the wounded gnaw at our conscience and are a reflection of our decision to wage war. We view these images from the Civil War and the effects of the Minie Ball with some emotional detachment afforded by the space of 150 years but seeing the mutilated soldiers from Iraq and Afghanistan evokes instant horror as these are our current brothers, sisters, fathers and mothers and the results of our own decisions.

While the photographs in this series do not show the internal havoc caused by these bullets the collection of shattered bones that Bontecou and others sent to the Army Medical Museum demonstrated their brutal effectiveness. Because of the shattered bones and infectious debris most surgeons amputated arms and legs so as to not to have the patient die from secondary infections.

Many of the men we see here are going to die. Some know it, others don't. Some were in the hospital for months undergoing surgeries and healing, hoping to live, right up to the time they acquired a hospital borne infection. Then quickly, quietly and stoically they died. The 1000+ photographs that Bontecou took reflect this entire experience of war. Bontecou's photographs documented the battle against gunshot wounds. His clinical photographs were a critical and necessary medical response to the threat of the Minie ball. A handful of other surgeons did send some photographs of their patients to the AMM but Bontecou meticulously documented the original wound, the complications, healed state or advanced effect of the wound prior to the soldiers death. He also supplied a written synopsis of treatment. They not only helped other surgeons, they established a tradition that would become the standard of documentation in following new or unusual war wounds.

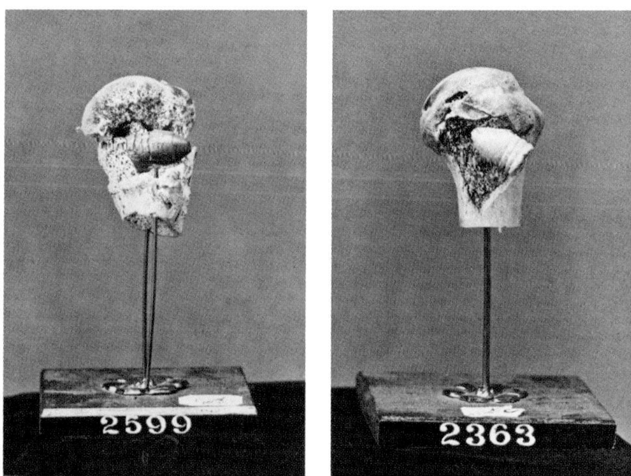

MINIE BALL BULLETS EMBEDDED IN BONES, BONTECOU SPECIMENS 2599 AND 2363.

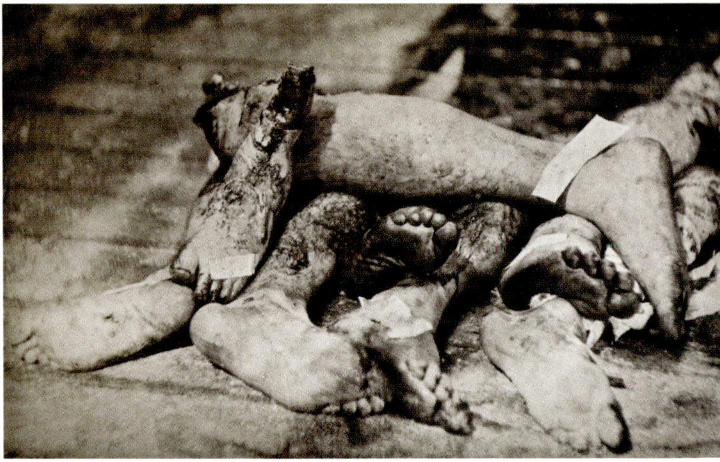

"A MORNING'S WORK" BONTECOU'S LABEL FOR HIS ICONIC IMAGE OF WARTIME LABORS.

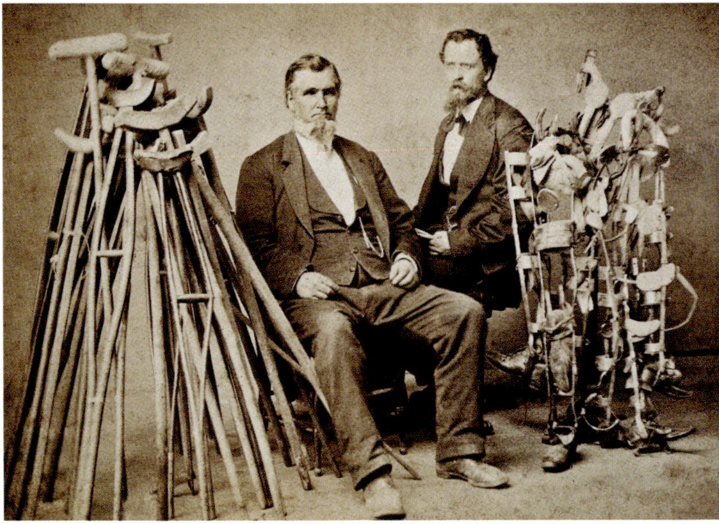

SALESMEN FOR PROSTHETIC APPLIANCES POSE WITH PILES OF THE DEVICES.

DEATH & SACRIFICE

The death of one man is a tragedy, the death of a million a statistic.
-Kurt Tucholsky, 1932, often attributed to Joseph Stalin

Bontecou's clinical photographs of soldiers bring to light the singular tragedies. These photographs also let us better comprehend the carnage of the 475,000 wounded. That figure does not adequately reflect the hundreds of thousands with disease that were not counted in the wounded casualty figures. Only those who died from disease were counted as casualties. Disease killed about three times as many as were killed in battle. About 3 million men fought in the war, 2.1 million for the Union and 700,000 for the Confederacy. About 75% of men of military age were engaged in the conflict. About 620,000 died, roughly one in four who fought. There were at least 50,000 civilian casualties. Union statistics list 360,000 dead, but only about 100,000 were by battle wounds, 260,000 were by disease. There were over 6 million reported instances of disease among Union soldiers. By 1865 the rate of diarrhea and dysentery was 995 per 1000 troops. The main deaths due to disease as recorded on sick reports were: 57,000 dead from diarrhea and dysentery, 45,000 from camp fevers (typho-malarial), 20,000 from pneumonia. Hundreds of thousands of soldiers survived the war with diseases that made their lives miserable and ultimately tens of thousands died from their maladies in the decade after the war. The enormity of the medical care required overwhelmed available resources. A good example is that when Union army regimental physicians left Gettysburg to follow the army for the next battle the remaining surgeons each had about 900 patients. The faces of Bontecou's patient's often reflect the situation of the time: fear, acceptance, stoicism, and resolve.

The essence of a Civil War soldier's duty was sacrifice. There was a very high chance of death, wounding or being maimed by disease. Chaplains often reminded the men at sermons that killing and dying was the soldier's duty. Soldiers knew about personal killing as battle lines were so close they could see the face of the man they shot or see the man next to them shot. Bayonet charges and hand-to-hand fighting further brought the act of killing directly into a soldier's reality. One watched as his friends, and at times relatives, received their death wound. Every battle had close encounter episodes. This was not a war fought at great distances but with tight shoulder-to-shoulder formations.

Although death was a constant companion, the soldier's greatest fear was loss of identity and his family not knowing what happened to him, or where he was buried. Unfortunately this was too often the case for the common soldier. ID tags could be bought but most soldiers before battle simply pinned their name on the inside of their uniform. It is amazing to us today that at the start of the Civil War there was no official responsibility on the part of the government to account for its servicemen. There was no requirement to notify a family of death or wounding, for identification of a soldier's body, or where he was buried. On every soldier's mind was the fear of being treated no differently than a farm animal, buried unidentified in a shallow grave where wild animals would feed on him. The wealthy made preparations with friends and family to retrieve their bodies. Others relied on death pacts with their fellow soldiers. Southern officers went into battle with their servants. The numbers of slaves accompanying Confederate armies was substantial, at Gettysburg an estimated 6,000 slaves were present. When the master died it was the slave's duty to retrieve his body and bring him home. Unfortunately, despite their best efforts, more than one-third of the 620,000 soldiers who died in the war were buried unidentified. About 175,000 of the Union graves after reburial in national cemeteries to this day are simply marked "unknown."

Soldier's thoughts about death are detailed in numerous letters, journals and pronouncements. Being out of a battle and being in a hospital did not take one out of harms way as "hospitalism" the deadly wound infections contracted in hospitals killed thousands—many after they thought they were secure. Others caught whatever epidemic disease that rampaged through their ward. Physicians and hospital personnel were among the victims. Several of Bontecou's assistant surgeons died in the epidemics at Harewood.

Years after the war Union Surgeon General Alexander Hammond, who created the Army Medical Museum, noted that the war was fought at "the end of the medical middle ages." It was two years after the war, in 1867, that Joseph Lister, MD announced his discovery of antiseptic surgical principles. It was not until 1883 that Robert Koch described the germ theory of disease. Until then infection remained an intriguing mystery, much like cancer is today. In the Civil War a small flesh wound could result in death from infection at anytime. Bontecou's photographs illustrate these deadly infections (pyemia, hospital gangrene, erysipelas) and show us soldiers whose lives would soon be snuffed out. Some of his photographs clearly illustrate the terrible conditions patients lived with and that physicians faced without the knowledge or tools to treat. Those who survived were marred and mentally scarred for life. While post traumatic stress syndrome (PTSS) is well recognized today, it was extremely common in those who experienced combat in the Civil War.

During and after the war, tens of thousands who experienced the battles, as well as hospitals and the dead and dying, almost as a chorus wrote that the suffering exceeded language and understanding. The verbal capacity to describe the horror and events was believed to be beyond expression. Upon the realization of the magnitude of the numbers killed and wounded, writers became obsessed with emphasizing the importance of the individual life. The one could be somebody's all. Bontecou's photographs are portraits that rivet our eyes to these individuals. It is always posited by governments that shared national loss and sacrifice transcends individual bereavements--yet these photographs take us back to that individual bereavement. In *Sleeping Beauty: Memorial Photography in America* I detailed the history of an American culture living with death as a result of disease. While epidemics killed millions during the century, the Civil War wreaked havoc on servicemen and ultimately their families. Personal sacrifice was a patriotic duty and personal grief was managed for the good of the nation. After the war, to better deal with the unprecedented deaths and loss, two ideologies rose to prominence in American culture. Consolation literature encouraged notions of an afterlife in an earth-like heaven. Elizabeth Phelp's *The Gates Ajar*, published in 1868, was the second most popular novel of the 19th century (*Uncle Tom's Cabin* was the first). Being reunited with a loved one after death was the critical theme. The other ideology was spiritualism, which posited that the dead still live but in a special heavenly space and they can communicate with the living through special communicators. These philosophies offered hope that the loss was not permanent. In reality, Americans lived with grief and loss for the rest of the century -- until the medical accomplishments of the 1890s offered conquest of disease and promise of a long healthy life.

For rest of their lives those who survived the war lived with the memory of their lost companions. The mutilated served as a constant reminder as to the human price of the war. In 1868 the first Decoration Day to honor the dead and give dignity to the survivors was established. May 30th was the day originally chosen as it was not the anniversary of a major battle. Now renamed Memorial Day, and made by law the last Monday in May, it has evolved into America's official national day of mourning for all those who died while in service to the nation. Drew Gilpin Faust, in his *This Republic of Suffering: Death and the American Civil War*, details the death, dying, and burying rituals associated with the Civil War and its aftermath, as well as the consolation and memorialization adjustments made after the war in response to the untimely death of over 670,000 citizens.

American Soldiers were ready to die and die honorably. By the nineteenth century the idea of the 'Good Death' was an American ideal and was a shared by all religious groups. People in this time period talked about death much the same as we today talk about the weather. *Ars moriendi* was the tradition of the art of dying, which dictated rules of conduct, most importantly how to give up ones soul "gladly and willingly." Sudden death in battle could preclude this noble act but once wounded, servicemen knew the traditions and how to behave. The many stories of mortally wounded soldiers and their last words and pronouncements were, and still are, the most heart rendering episodes of the conflict. Soldiers were dying in their "brother's" arms and didn't want to let them or society down. It was their duty to die for their country's noble cause, Union or Confederate, and do it honorably. Many servicemen transitioned from soldier to symbolic wounded, dying patriot. Modern audiences look on the faces of these wounded men pondering their pain, resolve and apparent stoicism. But we shouldn't forget that they were living in an age when death was part of everyday life in the American culture. The war was like another deadly epidemic simply taking at random your family and friends.

Dying in a hospital had some distinct advantages as the patient or a nurse (if the patient was not lucid) wrote home to his family during his stay so that the family knew where to retrieve the serviceman's body if he died. The Adams Express Company had established regulations for sanitary and safe transport of bodies and shipped tens of thousands home during the war. Wealthy families could afford embalming and special metal caskets were available to preserve the dead.

While a mass burial of American soldiers would seem outrageous today, at the time the thousands of wounded after a battle were the first concern, and overwhelmed medical ability to care for them. In many battles wounded were left suffering unattended on the battlefield for days. The task of carefully burying and recording the identity of the dead seemed unimportant as the wounded took precedence. As the war progressed, battles involved tens of thousands. At Antietam, on one day, Sept 17, 1862, 3850 were killed and 17,200 wounded. At Gettysburg over 7800 lay dead on the field along with over 3000 horses, about 27,000 were wounded. When regimental surgeons left with their units as the Union army prepared for the next battle, each remaining surgeon had about 900 patients to care for and ultimately place in general hospitals. It is not surprising, so little attention was paid to the dead.

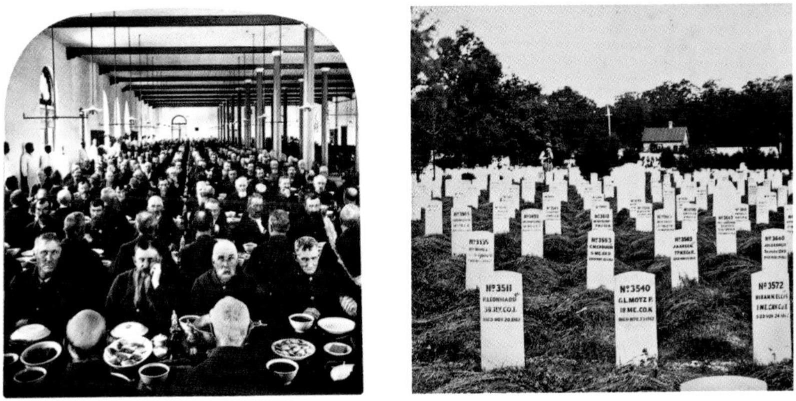

THE COST OF WAR. A) DISABLED SOLDIERS AT THE SOLDIERS HOME IN MARION INDIANA 1885. B) REBURIED BODIES AT A NEW NATIONAL CEMETERY. AN INTERESTING ASPECT IS THE GRAVES OF A LAUNDRESS AND TEAMSTER BURIED AMONG THE SOLDIERS—CIVILIANS WERE NOT LISTED IN THE COUNT OF MILITARY DEAD. THE CEMETERY PHOTO (PRODUCED ABOUT 1872) HAS ONLY IDENTIFIED GRAVES PROBABLY ISSUED TO SHOW THE GOVERNMENT'S ATTEMPT TO TAKE CARE OF THE DEAD.

Since hundreds of thousands of soldiers were buried unidentified, the anguish of surviving families who had undocumented, unconfirmed and unrecognized loss prompted government action. In 1862 the Union authorized payments to surviving widows and families. In 1864 Congress established a graves registration unit, which was not truly effective until after the war. Irrefutable evidence of the death of a loved one is necessary for emotional acceptance of loss. After the war businesses were established to identify remains and provide proper burial in the newly established national cemeteries, or if acceptable, return a body to the family.

Dying in a major general hospital offered a better chance of grave identification as surgeons had responsibility for hospital burial grounds. Hopefully the names of the deceased and where they were buried would be recorded. Several of Bontecou's photographs are labeled 'unidentified' and at the end of the war they served as potential identification records. Bontecou's images are a visual legacy of the war and also of soldiers' families. In many instances the only surviving photograph of an ancestor is the clinical image taken by Bontecou. Ted Karle, writing in *Military Images* magazine in 2007, described how he found his great grandfather, Peter Karle's nude photo taken by Bontecou in the National Archives.

During the war two organizations, the US Sanitary Commission and the Christian Commission, were established to assist servicemen, as the government was ill prepared for war or for providing for its servicemen. These organizations provided for many of the servicemen's basic needs. Their personnel also communicated with families, assisted the wounded and helped keep track of the dead. The Christian Commission documented 92,000 letters their staff wrote for the wounded and sick during the conflict. Private organizations such as Friends of Missing Men of the United Sates Army helped with grave location. Eventually the U.S. Sanitary Commission, an official government agency established to coordinate volunteer philanthropic efforts, became involved with burials and identification.

At the end of the war records officially listed only 101,736 registered Union burials. About 259,000 Union dead were in undocumented locations. With the war's end the Federal government sought to find the Union graves. In June 1865, the 1st US Volunteer Veterans Core was created and dispatched to bury only "Union" remains at the Wilderness Battlefield. They found thousands of skeleton parts and created a large pile of skulls, which were then buried 10 skulls to a coffin, with bones used as fill. Union soldiers graves in Confederate states were regularly obliterated. In February 1866 a Military general order forbade the desecration of Union graves. In 1867 a new era of federal obligation was established as Congress passed legislation for re-internment of all Union dead to local and newly established national cemeteries. The Confederate dead were left to the responsibility of Southern civilian organizations such as the Association of Southern Mothers. It cost about $9.75 each to move the Federal bodies and when the program ended in 1871, 303,536 Union soldiers were reburied in 74 national cemeteries. Only 54% of the men were identified. In 1898 government responsibility for Confederate dead was assumed. With that act, the dead of the Civil War became not Union or Confederate dead but America's dead. 620,000 individuals lost in creating the modern Union. The staggering loss became one powerful force of change, as millions of families were effected. It compelled the government to accept responsibility for all its servicemen. One major social legacy of the Civil War was the government recognition of the obligation to a service person's family if they died on duty. Grasping the meaning of a single death, and the meaning of hundreds of thousands, illustrates war's magnitude helped by poignant pictures of individuals. Mass death is unintelligible whereas focusing on one death allows us to better understand the tragedy.

THE FINAL BATTLES

The Civil War, April 1861-April 1865, was America's bloodiest war, with over 1,100,000 military casualties. A largely overlooked aspect of the war is the civilian casualties. Perhaps more than 50,000 civilians died including contraband, other blacks, southern and border state citizens and northern civilians caught in the battlefields, which included towns and villages. There were 10,055 battles and skirmishes of which 391 are considered major battles. The turning point of the war was early July, 1863. At the Battle of Gettysburg (July 1-3), Major General George Meade, stopped Lee's advance into the North. And on July 4, 1863, Major General Ulysses S. Grant's brilliant siege and battle strategy captured Vicksburg, Mississippi. With Vicksburg's fall Lt. General John Pemberton surrendered his army of 24,000 Confederates. This victory in the Mississippi campaign, in the "Western Theatre" of war, effectively split the Confederacy in two and opened the way for more Union victories. Grant's brilliance and aggressive actions won him the admiration of President Lincoln and he was appointed Lt. General and then in 1864 to a position only George Washington had previously held, General-in-Chief of the Army. He was then directed to lead the Army of the Potomac in the East to fight General Robert E. Lee's Army of Northern Virginia. The lack of initiative and indecisiveness of prior Union Generals had lost numerous opportunities to put an end to the conflict. Grant's aggressive determination to never retreat and constantly fight would bring the bloody conflict to its end.

Grant's role in the East began at the Battle of the Wilderness on May 5, 1864 and culminated in Lee's surrender on April 9, 1865. To put this in perspective for modern war historians the time period mimics that of the American action in the WWII European war. The Allies landed in France on D-Day, June 6, 1944 and the European war ended on May 8, 1945. In both wars those 11 months were hellish. The great majority of Dr. Bontecou's photographs were from the battles during this last time period of the war. May 1864-April 9, 1865. Over half of these photographs were from battles during the last days of the war, March 25 to April 9, 1865.

The first battles of Grant's sustained offensive against Lee's Army of Northern Virginia are known as the Overland Campaign. The major episodes were the battles of the Wilderness (May 5-7, 1864), Spotsylvania Court House (May 8-21, 1864), and Cold Harbor (May 31-June 12, 1864). Grant believed the key to victory was constant unrelenting pressure against all Confederate forces even if in some battles he suffered great losses. At Cold Harbor on June 3rd over 7,000 Union troops were killed or wounded in about 30 minutes. It was a major Confederate victory. However, Grant did not stop his armies and continued to move toward Richmond and its guardian city, Petersburg. Petersburg, located near Richmond, Virginia, the capital of the Confederacy, was the site of all-important Southern railroad junctions. The city was the last obstacle to capturing Richmond and was well fortified. Grant hoped to close off this transportation terminus, which had kept the city of Richmond and Lee's troops supplied.

After a series of battles around Petersburg, by June 18th Grant was facing well-entrenched rebel troops. Grant's strategy of a campaign of attrition would ultimately crush the Confederacy. The North, like the United States in WWII, had become an industrialized war machine with new weapons and soldiers. New York State alone had more industrial capacity than the entire Confederacy. The Siege of Petersburg (June 1864 to March 1865) was a stalemate and an impending disaster for Lee as Grant extended his battle lines. During the early siege, on July 30th, 1864, a potentially brilliant idea on the part of the Union forces turned into a fiasco. Pennsylvania miners dug tunnels under Confederate positions and exploded four tons of gunpowder, hoping to create a breach in the rebel defenses. Then in the last hours, the men who had been trained to lead the attack – US Colored Troops units--were replaced by inexperienced units of white troops. It was a slaughter. Confederate troops regrouped and had a turkey shoot as they lined the crater and shot at the men trapped inside who were supposed to go around it. Smaller battles continued around Petersburg for months as the siege intensified.

The last battles of the assault at Petersburg (March 25-April 2), and Appomattox Campaign Battles (April 3-April 9, 1865) are designated the Petersburg-Appomattox Campaigns. Grant's strategy was brilliant. With hundreds of thousands of men at his disposal he kept on extending his battle lines to 30 miles trying to outflank the Confederates. At the beginning of the siege he had about 100,000 men to Lee's 55,000. His army expanded as Lee's contracted. Lee dreaded a siege as it denied him mobility and he couldn't send troops to help other armies fighting in the Western Theater against Major General William Sherman. This entrenchment of Lee's major forces gave time for Sherman's armies to continue the "march to the sea" and devastate Georgia and South Carolina. By March 21, 1865 Sherman had conquered major rebel forces in North Carolina and could send his army to Virginia to augment Grants.

Direct frontal attacks against Lee's entrenched forces were repulsed each time and the engineering ingenuity of the trench system presaged those of World War I.

Small Union attempts to find weaknesses in the line were unrewarding and artillery duels became common. As the Petersburg line stretched, Lee's inadequate forces were continually thinned. Several strategic strongholds called 'forts' were created by Federal and Confederate troops in front of Petersburg. Heavy artillery, infantry, and other units manned these fortified installations. Physical obstacles were extensive and included rows of deep trenches, wooden spikes and other impediments. Major battles were hardly ever fought in winter and Lee knew time was running out. Not waiting to be overrun or be out-flanked, he concentrated about 12,000 of his best troops for one great attack. On March 25, 1865, Lee launched a surprise attack against Grant's central position, Fort Steadman the foremost Federal installation. His idea was to split the Federal line and break the impending encirclement. While the attack was at first successful, it ultimately failed. Grant seized the opportunity and launched major offensives. On April 1st and 2nd a Federal attack at nearby Five Forks, a major crossroads, broke the Confederate ranks. Petersburg and then Richmond were captured. Rail lines and supplies were captured in battles at Sayler's Creek. Another series of food and artillery wagons were captured by cavalry led by General George Armstrong Custer. One train that was to bring food to Lee's starving army contained ammunition. After a series of battles at Farmville, Hatcher's Run, Amelia Court House, and Appomattox, with his army's food and supplies captured, the rail lines in Union hands, and his remaining men exhausted, Lee surrendered on April 9, 1865.

Bontecou's photographs include servicemen from all the major battles of Grant's final campaigns. The great majority of the images are from the last days of the war. The details of these battles are represented profusely on the internet and in numerous books, so a detailed description of the action and units involved can be easily found.

Reed Bontecou produced the largest number of clinical photographs made during the Civil War, representing the majority of the war images. The photographs were taken mainly between May, 1864 and July, 1865. After the war he personally assembled the images into four albums. The first was his unique CdV album. Along with the 570 images are a list of 82 assistant surgeons, military papers and hospital record cards. The second and third albums were a two volume set each with over 100 5 ½ by 7 ½ photographs mounted with text printed on the backs.. The fourth album was a compilation of about 120 mounted 5 ½ by 7 ½ inch images of his photographs mixed with those taken at the AMM. This compilation album includes diagrams with drawings of suspected bullet paths on the photographs of GSW patients. All of these albums have personal notations signed by Bontecou and all are in the Burns Collection.

Starting in late 1864 Bontecou began sending packets of photographs to the AMM. In a letter dated March 1866, he sends a packet of CdVs to the AMM and asked that they not be bound into albums yet as he "had more to send" and "Please have the album marked 'contributed'." The AMM staff wrote on the letter, "valuable contribution of photographs." One of the photographs from this packet, with the SGO stamp of March 21, 1866, is shown on page 7. The AMM lists in 1866 four CdV volumes donated by Bontecou of 364, 58, 65, and 66 "surgical cases." Only 17 of these early donated photographs remain in the museum. In 1866-1869 Bontecou donated hundreds of more images. The contributed photographs over number 899 were not his CdV prints but his large oval photographs produced after the war. Of the several hundred contributed photographs Bontecou donated to the museum only 230 remain at the AMM, most above number 898, as the others were dispersed by Dr. Daniel Lamb in the early 20th century. Still in the collection are numbers 898 through 1108, all but five of these by Bontecou. Civil War images at the AMM runs to number 1604. The photographic exchange worked both ways as negatives were reprinted by the AMM for Bontecou and sent to him. In a letter dated Sept 25, 1866 he writes about "not receiving mounted views of the Wilderness and some from the negatives I left with 'Bell.' There were about ten or twelve whole size negatives of wounded men at 'Harewood' that had not been printed that I particularly desire." In a letter dated January 3, 1867 he writes about not getting recognition for a recent delivery of photographs. In Jan. 1869, he received 3 packets of photographs from the museum.

The CdV album was created after the war, as indicated by the presence of multiple alphabetical groupings of similar wound subjects with matching discharge dates.

The chronologically ordered dates of when patients were discharged, is the key to the time frame of assemblage. The album was compiled mostly from images taken and printed during the war and the images were part of the original hospital records of the patients. The hand-written notes on the front of many of the images showing operative scenes and pictures of fresh pathological specimens, as well as the death of patients, clearly place the time frame of the photographs as having been taken during the war. Many of these photographs are unique. A few of the patients depicted at the end of the album were transferred to Harewood in the fall of 1865 after other Washington DC hospitals closed; the photographs were taken at Harewood. On the back of the CdV pages is a hand written synopsis of the patient's history. A good number of photographs in the larger albums also have unique variant images in the CdV album. Over 200 regimental units are represented in the album.

There are several distinct clinical visual presentations in the album:

1. Patients with ID boards in the posing tradition of the master photographers
2. Posing without ID boards
3. Patients in bed and multiple patient images
4. Operative and specimen photographs

This volume, the first of several, depicts wounded men of about 101 Regiments holding identification chalkboards photographed in a vertical format. The chalkboards identify the soldier, his military unit, and often have the hospital record number. The next volume will depict poses without placards. The images of men not holding boards are the most artistic of Bontecou's photographs. Without the boards he could artistically pose his subjects to best show their wounds or disability. The next book in this CdV series will contain images of surgery, severe wounds, pathological specimens and other interesting images. A text emphasizing the large 5 ½ by 7 ½ inch portraits will be presented in *Final Harvest: The Civil War Photographs of Reed Bontecou.*

The photographic plates are arranged alphabetically by states but they are not presented in numerical order by unit. They are arranged by artistic merit and interest. As an aid for researchers two tables are presented. In one, the photographs have been arranged by state and listed in numerical order of regiment. The second table lists the soldiers in the battle in which they were wounded. Almost all the wounded shown in this text survived.

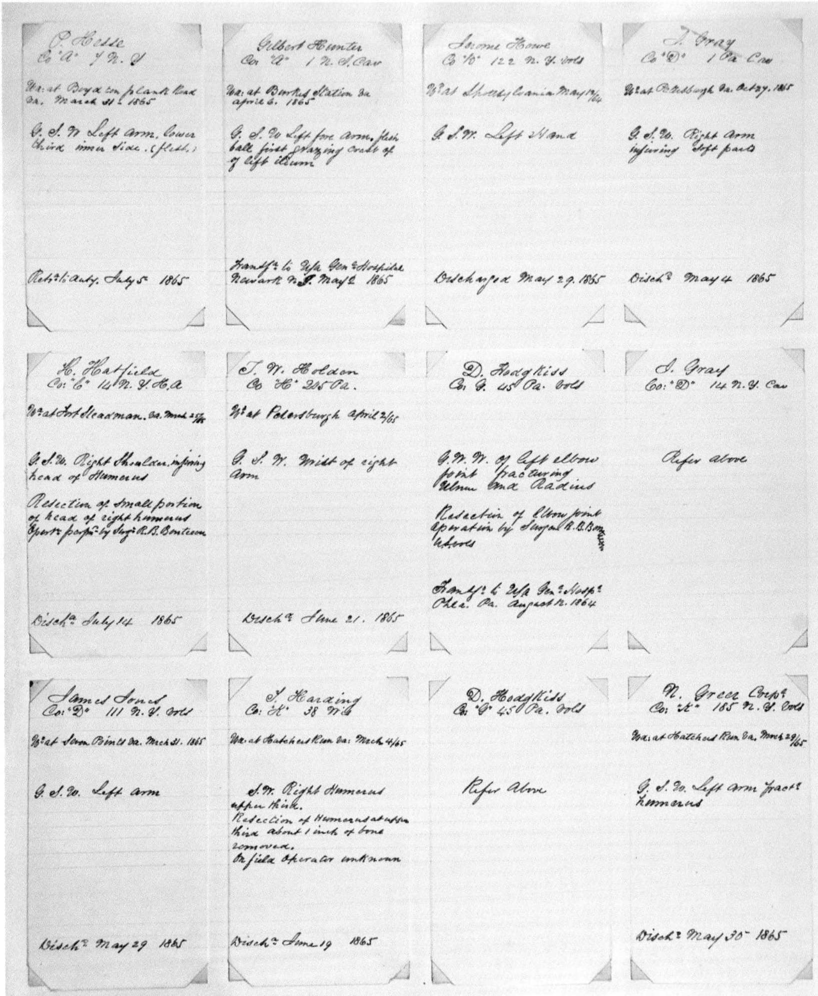

C. Hesse
Co. "A" 7 N. J.
Wd. at Boydton plank Road Va. March 31st 1865
G. S. W. Left arm, lower third inner side. (flesh.)
Retd. to duty. July 5th 1865

Gilbert Hunter
Co. "A" 1 N. J. Cav
Wd. at Burkes Station Va April 6. 1865
G. S. W. Left fore arm, flesh ball first grazing crest of of left ilium
Transf. to U.S.A. Gen. Hospital Newark N. J. May 2 1865

Jerome Howe
Co. "B" 122 N. Y. Vols
Wd. at Spottsylvania May 12/64
G. S. W. Left Hand
Discharged May 29. 1865

J. Gray
Co. "D" 1 Pa. Cav
Wd. at Petersburgh Va. Oct 27. 1865
G. S. W. Right arm injuring soft parts
Disch. May 4 1865

H. Hatfield
Co. "C" 14 N. Y. H. A
Wd. at Fort Steadman. Va. March 25/65
G. S. W. Right Shoulder, injuring head of Humerus
Resection of small portion of head of right humerus Opert. perfd. by Surg. R. B. Bontecou
Disch. July 14 1865

J. W. Holden
Co. "H" 205 Pa.
Wd. at Petersburgh April 2/65
G. S. W. Wrist of right arm
Disch. June 21. 1865

D. Hodgkiss
Co. G. 45 Pa. Vols
G. S. W. of left elbow joint fracturing Ulna and Radius
Resection of Elbow joint Operation by Surgeon R. B. Bontecou U.S. Vols
Transf. to U.S.A. Gen. Hosp. Phila. Pa. August 12. 1864

J. Gray
Co. "D" 14 N. Y. Cav
Refer above

James Jones
Co. "D" 111 N. Y. Vols
Wd. at Seven Points Va. March 31. 1865
G. S. W. Left arm
Disch. May 29 1865

J. Harding
Co. "K" 38 W. S.
Wd. at Hatchers Run Va. March 4/65
S. W. Right Humerus upper third.
Resection of Humerus at upper third about 1 inch of bone removed.
On field Operator unknown
Disch. June 19 1865

D. Hodgkiss
Co. "G" 45 Pa. Vols
Refer Above

N. Greer Corpl.
Co. "K" 185 N. Y. Vols
Wd. at Hatchers Run Va. March 29/65
G. S. W. Left arm fract. humerus
Disch. May 30 1865

EACH PHOTOGRAPH HAD AN EXPLANATION ON REVERSE. SOME HAD NOTATIONS ON THE IMAGE ITSELF, OTHERS PHOTOS WERE COMPLETE WITH A HOSPITAL RECORD CARD.

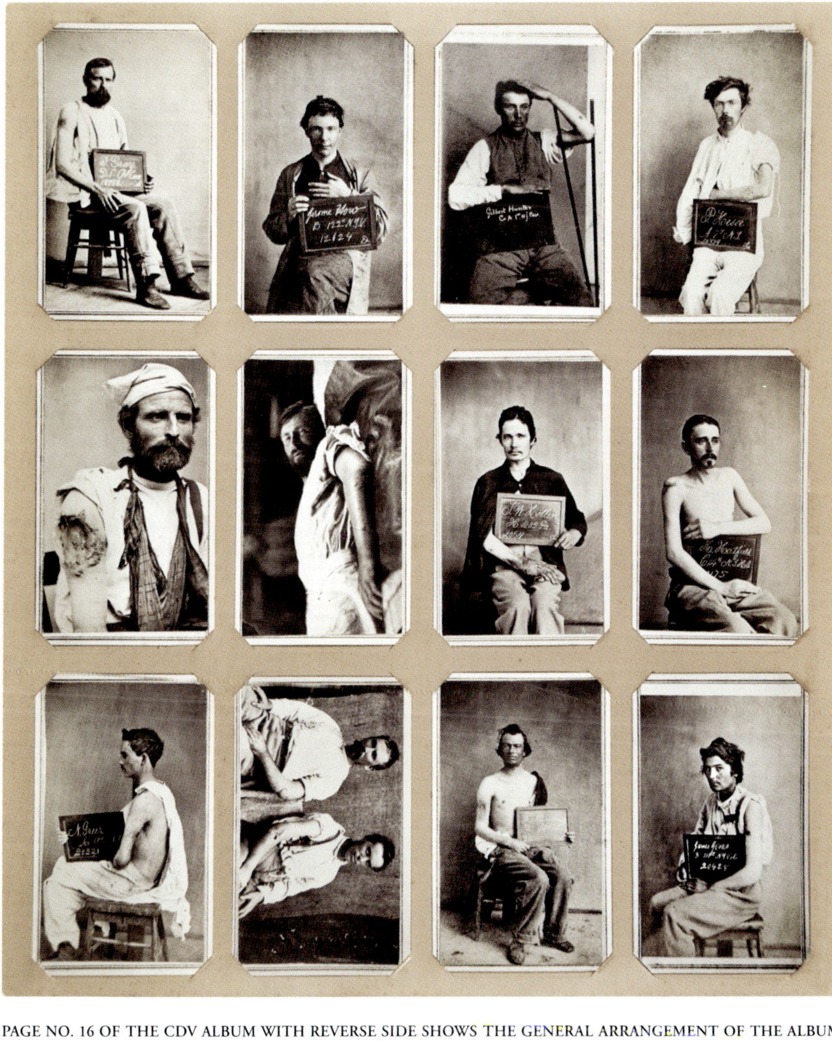

PAGE NO. 16 OF THE CDV ALBUM WITH REVERSE SIDE SHOWS THE GENERAL ARRANGEMENT OF THE ALBUM. THIS PAGE SHOWS HAND AND ARM WOUNDS OF SOLDIERS WITH LAST NAMES FROM G TO J.

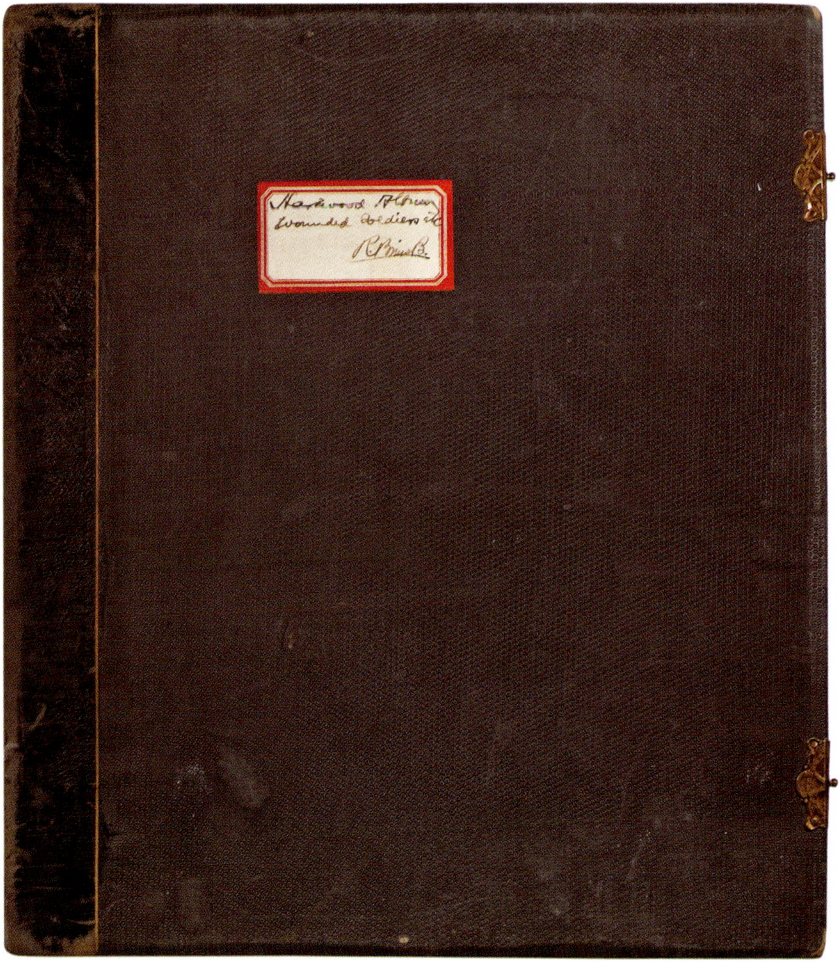

"HAREWOOD ALBUM, WOUNDED SOLDIERS, ETC." BONTECOU'S CARTE DE VISITE ALBUM.

THE REGIMENTS

CONFEDERATES

REG.	PLATE
8 LA	2
1 SC	1

SPECIAL UNITS

REG.	PLATE
2 Bat Vrc	5
4 US Inf	3
10 Vrc	7
31 US Col	4
10 Vrc	6

CONNECTICUT

REG.	PLATE
14 CT	8

DELAWARE

REG.	PLATE
1 DE	9

ILLINOIS

REG.	PLATE
26 IL	11
39 IL	10
111 IL	12

MAINE

REG.	PLATE
1 ME Cav	14
1 ME HA	15
4 ME Bat	16
11 ME	13

MARYLAND

REG.	PLATE
2 MD	18
7 MD	17

MASSACHUSETTS

REG.	PLATE
11 MA Bat	21
21 MA	20
37 MA	19
58 MA	22

MICHIGAN

REG.	PLATE
1 MI Cav	23
1 MI	27
5 MI	24
5 MI Cav	26
26 MI	25

NEW HAMPSHIRE

REG.	PLATE
1 NH	BC
2 NH	31
5 NH	28
6 NH	30
13 NH	29

NEW JERSEY

REG.	PLATE
1 NJ Cav	34
7 NJ	33
8 NJ	35
15 NJ	32

NEW YORK

REG.	PLATE
1 NY Cav	58
2 NY Cav	45
2 NY Ha	63
4 NY Ha	39
7 NY	71
8 NY Ha	69
9 NY Cav	48
10 NY Zou	36
14 NY Ha	59
15 NY Ha	62
24 NY Cav	64
42 NY	60
46 NY	37,38
52 NY	52

NEW YORK

REG.	PLATE
56 NY	57
64 NY	47
65 NY	68
69 NY	42
69 NY	70
79 NY Ha	FP
86 NY	40
94 NY	43
95 NY	50
106 NY	41
111 NY	61
120 NY	55
122 NY	54
124 NY	65
125 NY	53
151 NY	44
154 NY	56
155 NY	66
164 NY	51
185 NY	49
188 NY	67
188 NY	46

OHIO

REG.	PLATE
23 OH	73
126 OH	74
174 OH	72

PENNSYLVANIA

REG.	PLATE
1 PA Cav	86
8 PA Cav	92
17 PA Cav	87
48 PA	81
53 PA	75

PENNSYLVANIA

REG.	PLATE
61 PA	77
69 PA	78
87 PA	76
93 PA	84
116 PA	FC
148 PA	85
150 PA Mus	83
183 PA	82
191 PA	79
198 PA	80
200 PA	90
205 PA	88
207 PA	89
208 PA	91

RHODE ISLAND

REG.	PLATE
2 RI	94
7 RI	93

VERMONT

REG.	PLATE
1 VT Cav	96
11 VT	95

WEST VIRGINIA

REG.	PLATE
2 WV Cav	97

WISCONSIN

REG.	PLATE
5 WI	102
5 WI	100
6 WI	98
7 WI	99
38 WI	101

KEY: INFANTRY: INF. CAVALRY: CAV, HEAVY ARTILLERY: HA, UNITED STATES COLORED TROOPS: US COL, VETERAN'S RESERVE CORPS: VRC, VOLUNTEER: VOL, ZOUAVE: ZOU, BATTERY: BAT, MUSICIAN: MUS.

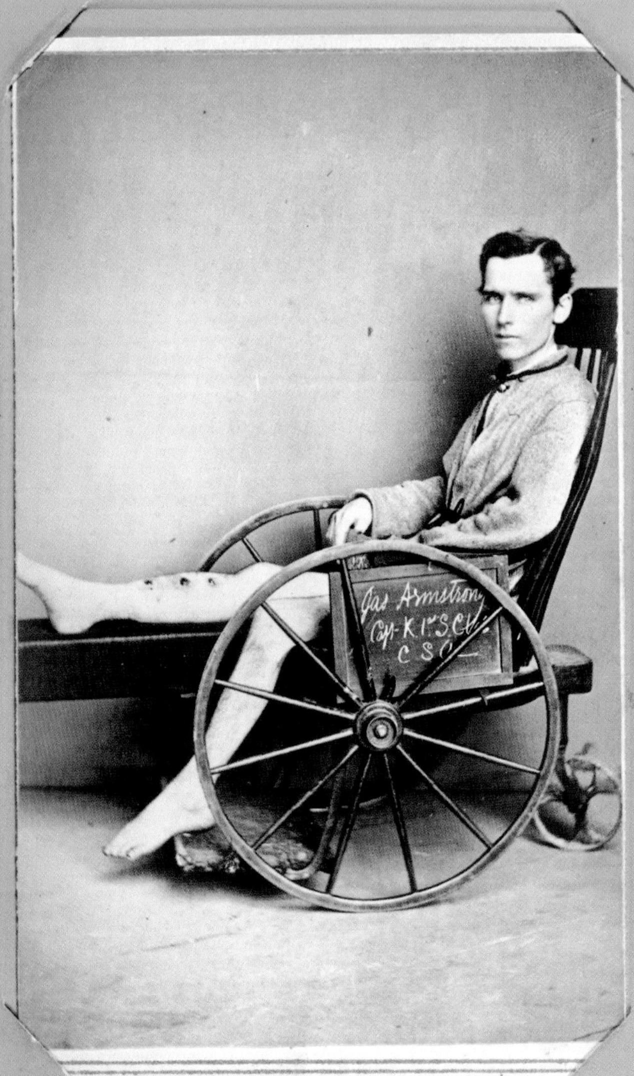

CONFEDERATES

JAS ARMSTRONG
CO K 1 SOUTH CAROLINA

PETERSBURG
APRIL 2, 1865

GSW RIGHT LEG,
FRACTURING THE TIBIA.

Aged 28, was admitted to HH, Sept.13, 1865. Partially convalescent from GSW through head of the humorous, ball passing through, shattering head of humorous. Wounded April 2nd at Battle of Petersburg. On admission the constitutional state of patient and condition of injured parts were tolerantly good; wounds still discharging pus and small fragments of dead bone. No operation was performed in this case. Nature to take its course. Patient is able to be about but he has no use of left arm, prospects of having a good and useful limb are very favorable. Articular surfaces of the shoulder joint not injured.

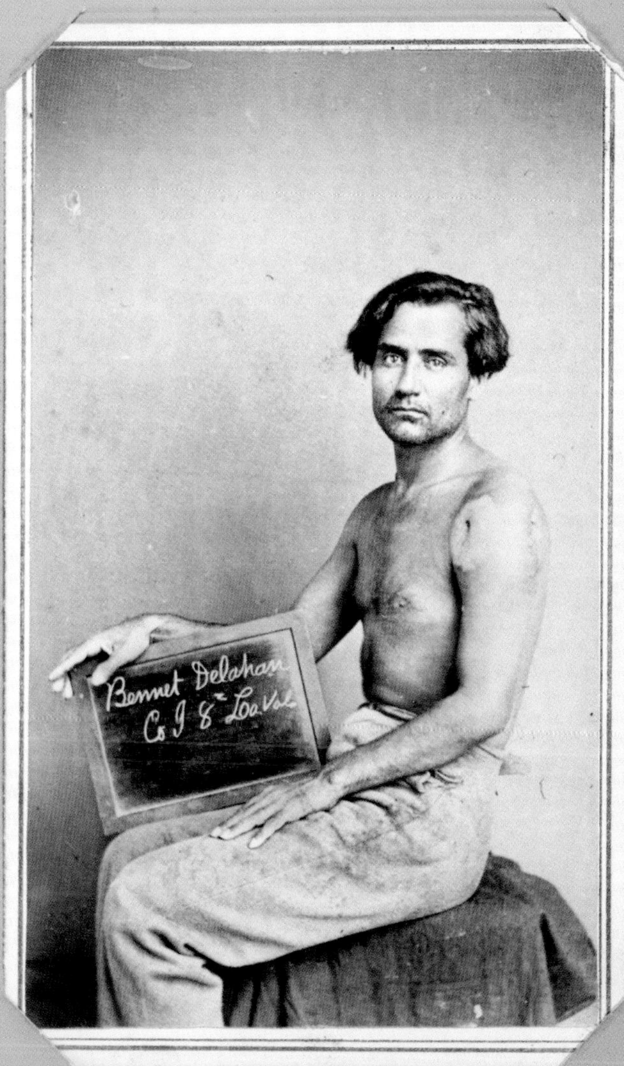

BENNET DELAHAN

CO J 8 LOUISIANA

PETERSBURG

APRIL 2, 1865

GSW LEFT SHOULDER. BALL PASSED THROUGH AND SHATTERD HEAD OF LEFT HUMEROUS.

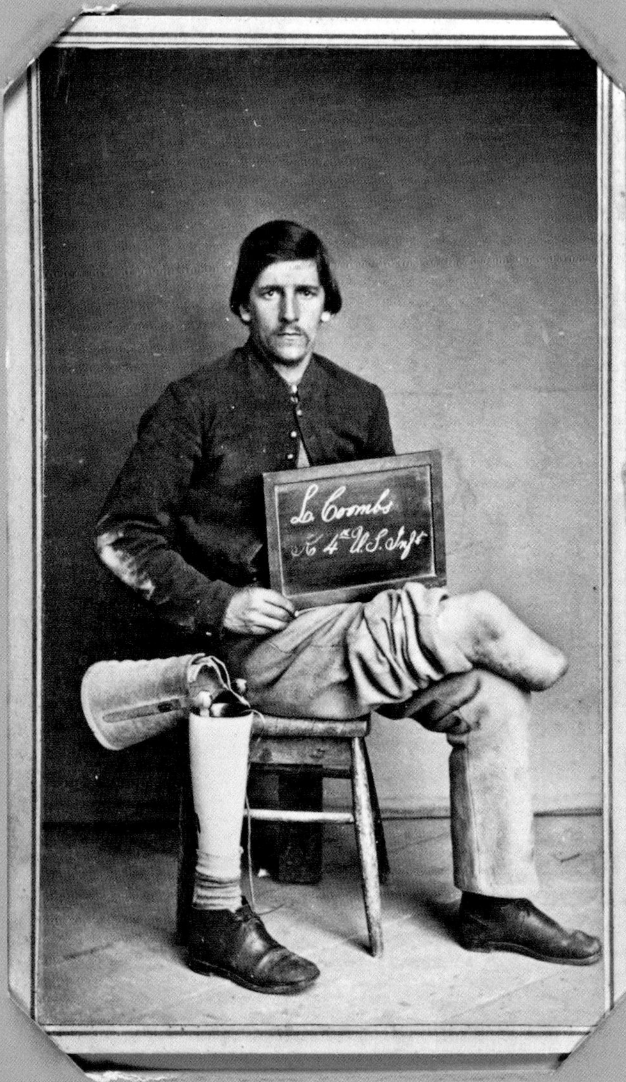

SPECIAL UNITS

LEVI COOMBS
CO K 4 US INF

NORTH ANNA RIVER
MAY 24, 1864

GSW, RIGHT LEG.
AMPUTATION OF RIGHT LEG.

DISCHARGED NOV 11, 1865

Pvt. Harris, 24 years old, was born in Lockhart, New York. He was in one of the black troop regiments that were specially trained to attack Confederate forces after the explosion that resulted in in what was to be known as the Battle of the Crater. Unfortunately, the trained US Colored Troop regiments were side lined from the planned course of action and were later employed to became part of the fiacso that resulted from the change of plans. Bontecou photographed five of these USCT men. In the 31st regiment, 54 were wounded, 31 killed and 14 MIA.

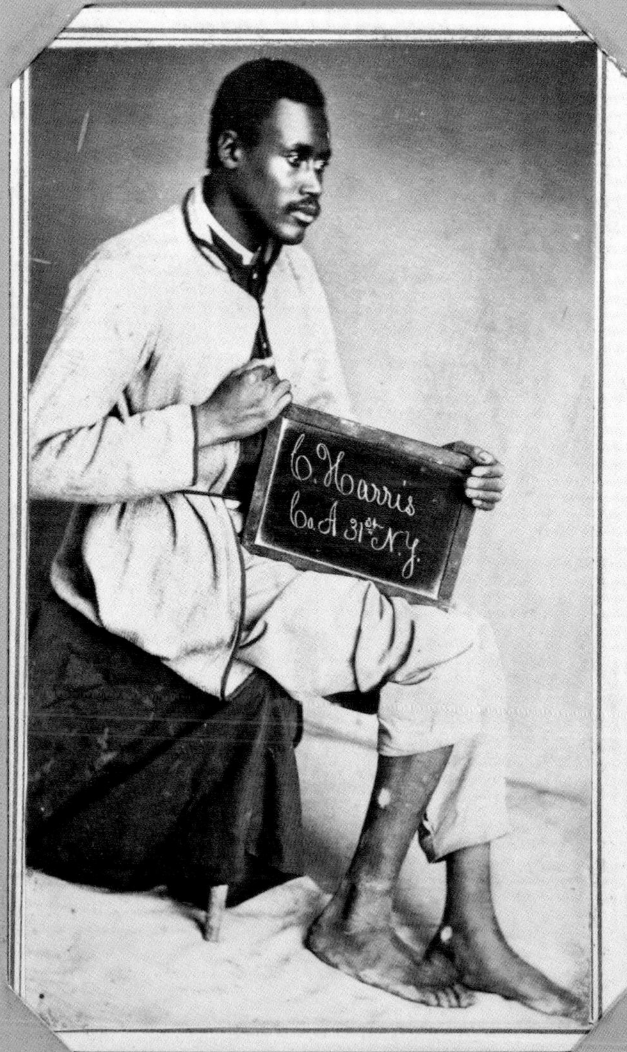

CHARLES HARRIS

CO A 31 US COL. TROOPS (NEW YORK)

PETERSBURG (BATTLE OF THE CRATER) JULY 30, 1864

GSW, RIGHT LEG & LEFT ANKLE.

DISCHARGED DEC 1, 1865

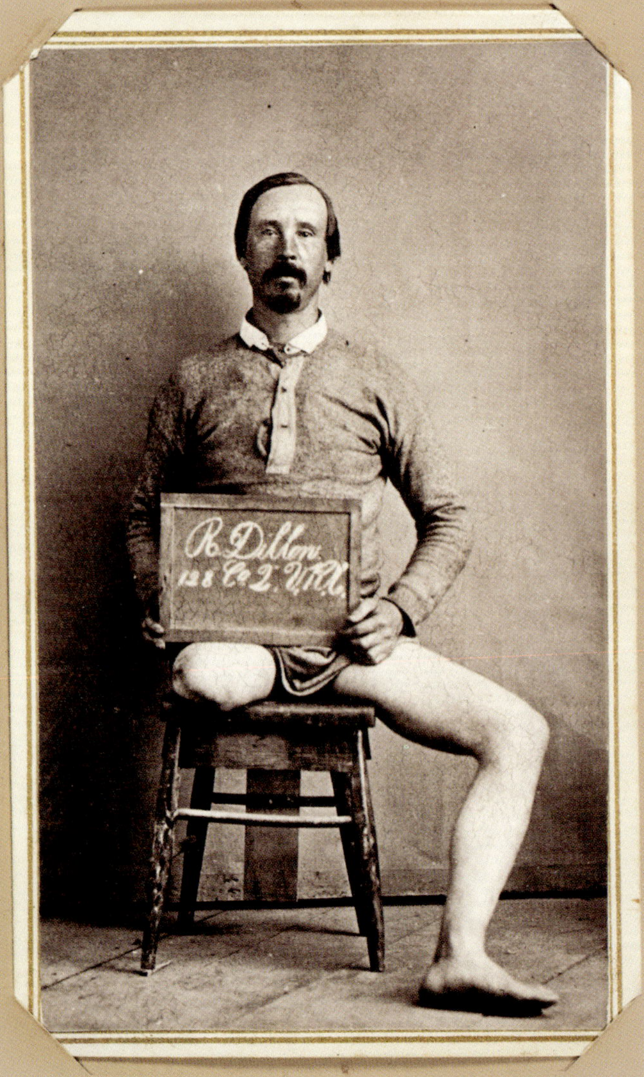

R. DILLON
2 BATTERY VRC

PETERSBURG
(BATTLE OF THE CRATER)
JULY 30, 1864

GSW RIGHT THIGH.
AMPUTATION OF RIGHT LEG.

DANIEL RICH
CO C 10 VRC
EX CO B 55 PA

GSW STERNUM

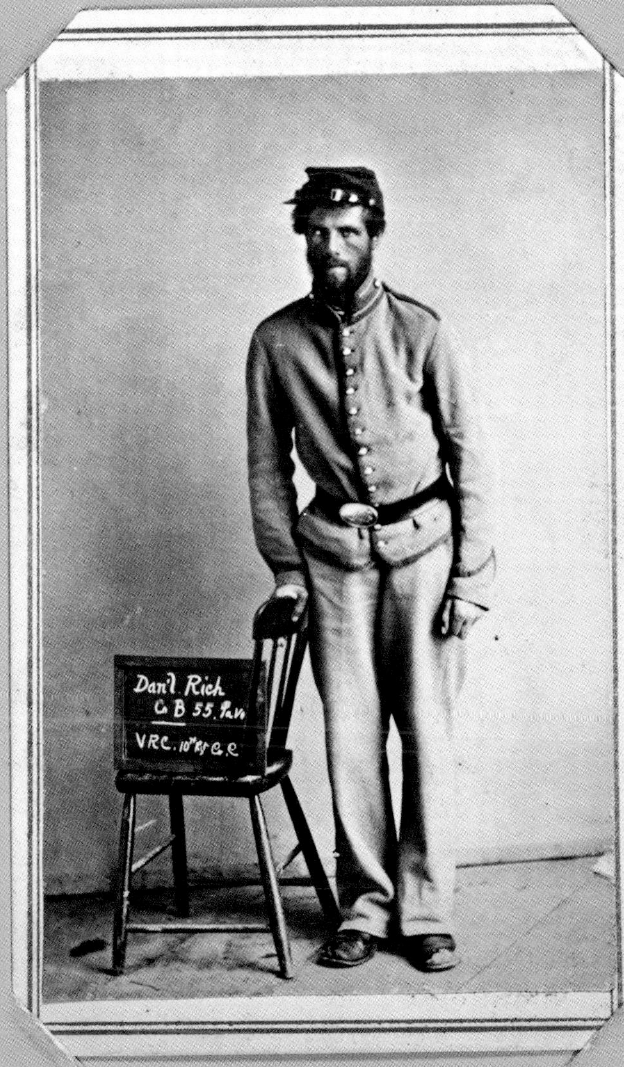

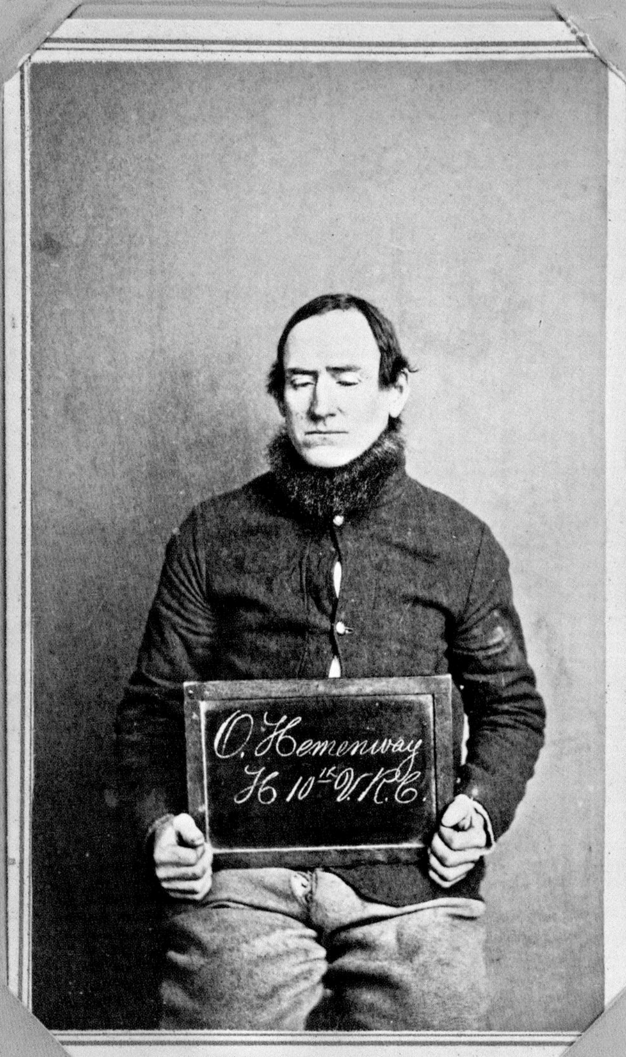

OTIS HEMENWAY

CO H 10 VRC

TOTAL LOSS OF VISION IN EYES DUE TO INFLAMATION CONTRACTED WHILE WITH HIS COMPANY AT CAMP.

DISCHARGED NOV 18, 1865

CONNECTICUT

MICHAEL DORSEY

CO D 14 CONN

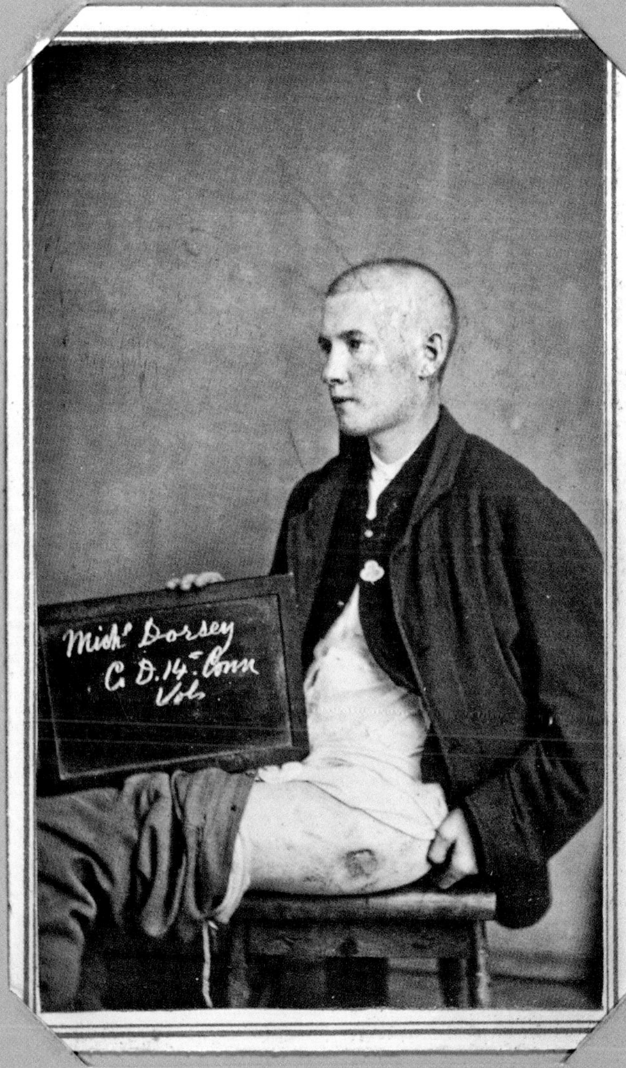

TYPHIOD FEVER.
(WITH ULCER)

DISCHARGED SEP 6, 1865

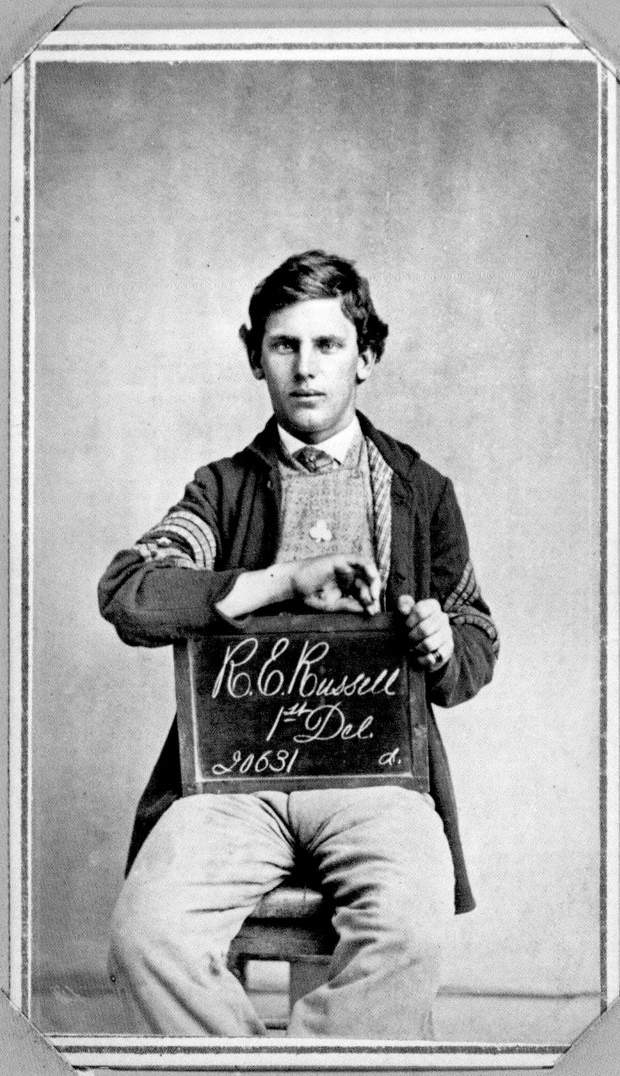

DELAWARE

R.E. RUSSELL

1 DEL

HATCHER'S RUN

APRIL 1, 1865

GSW, RIGHT HAND.
AMPUTATION OF MIDDLE
FINGER ON THE FIELD.

Aged 27, was admitted to HH, April 1, 1865, with gunshot wound to the left side of scalp, denuding skull. Wounded April 1, 1865, with a conoidal ball in action during the last charge before entering Petersburg, Va. Progress favorable. Transferred.

He had a head wound and also had an amputation of the right arm at the shoulder. By 1887 he was a patient in the Kansas State Insane Asylum. He had epilepsy, delusions and was homicidal and suicidal." His father was a physician.

ILLINOIS

E.O. VAN VALKENBURGH

CO C 39 IL

PETERSBURG

APRIL 1, 1865

GSW LEFT SIDE OF SCALP

TRANSFERRED MAY, 5 1865:

MADISON, WISCONSIN

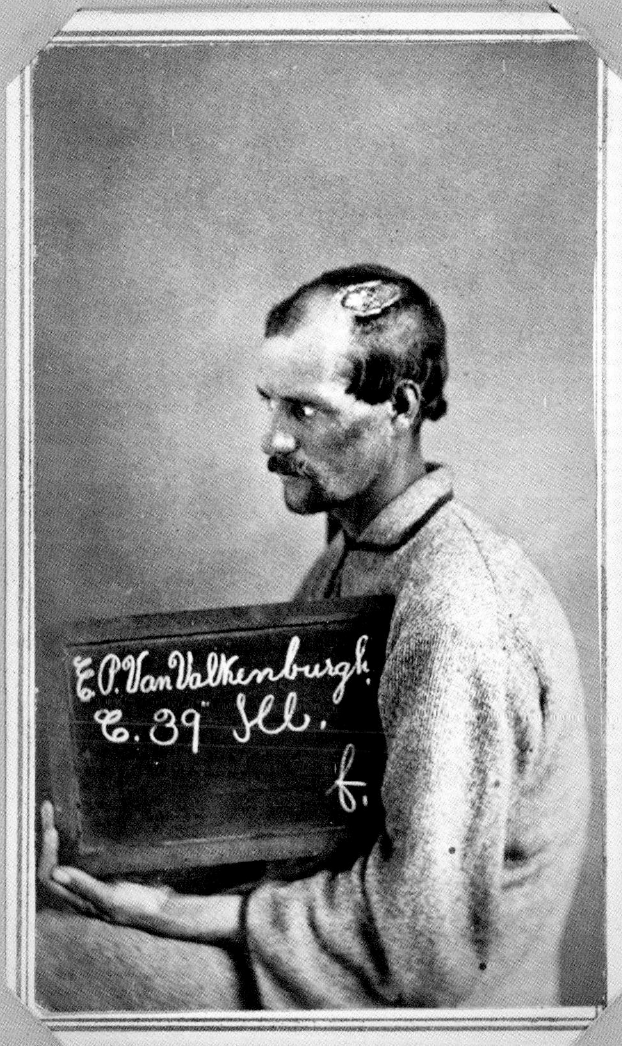

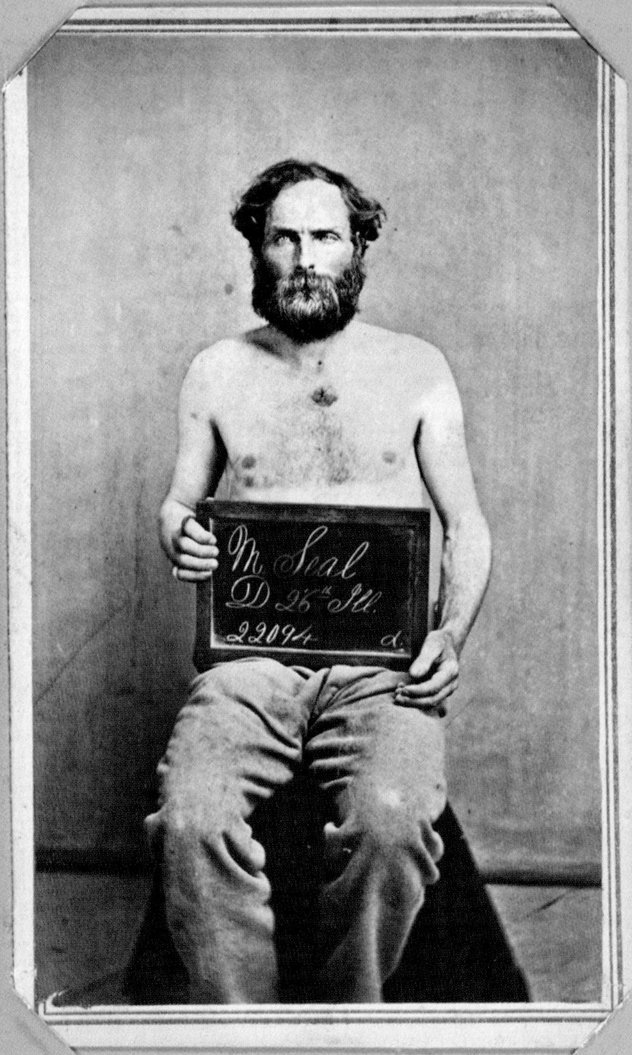

M. SEAL
CO D 26 ILL

GSW CHEST.
VARICOCELE.

DISCHARGED JULY 24, 1865

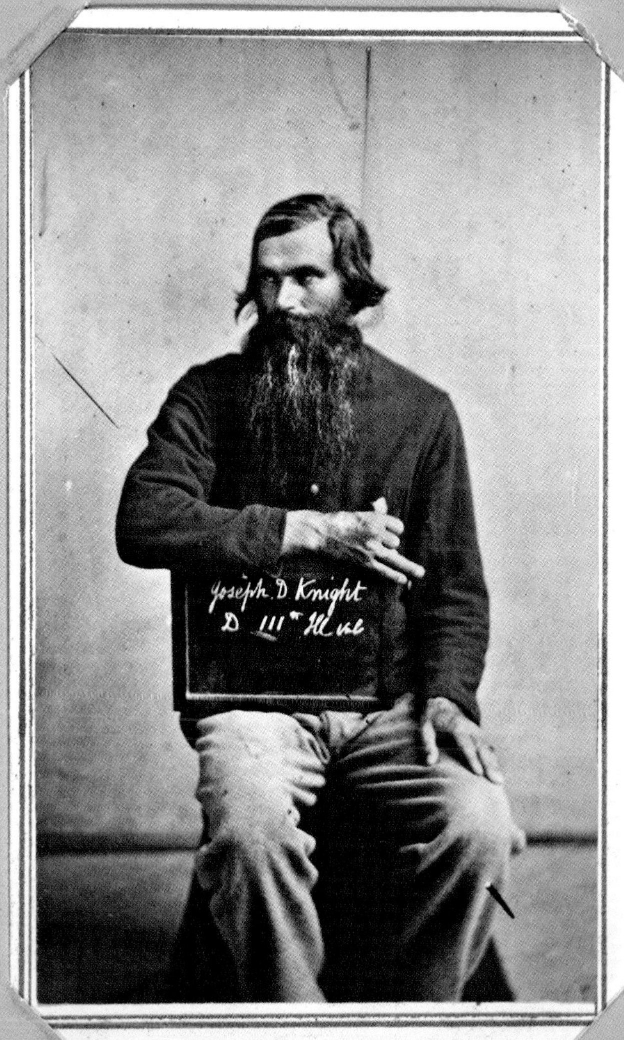

JOSEPH D. KNIGHT

CO D 111 ILL

MOSCOW, TN
FEBRUARY 14, 1863

GSW, LEFT & RIGHT HANDS. AMPUTATION OF FIRST & SECOND FINGER ON RIGHT.

DISCHARGED JULY 5, 1865

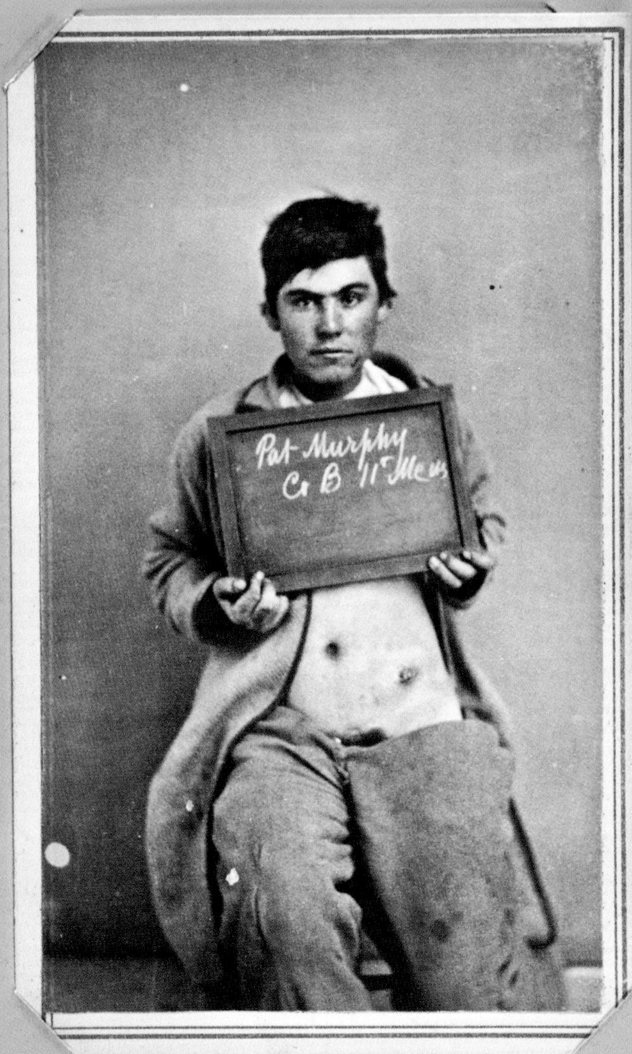

MAINE

PAT MURPHY
CO B 11 ME

PETERSBURG
APRIL 2, 1865

GSW, LEFT ILIAC REGION.

DISCHARGED JULY 8, 1865

34 years old. Died of dysentery while a prisoner of war at Andersonville, Georgia, July 21, 1864. Parker was captured at Old Church VA on March 2, 1864. Bontecou took this photograph when he was a patient at Harewood. Parker's case is a good example of the extreme physical condition under which soldiers were considered fit for duty.

AARON PARKER

CO D 1 ME CAV

CHRONIC DIARRHEA.

DIED JULY 21, 1864

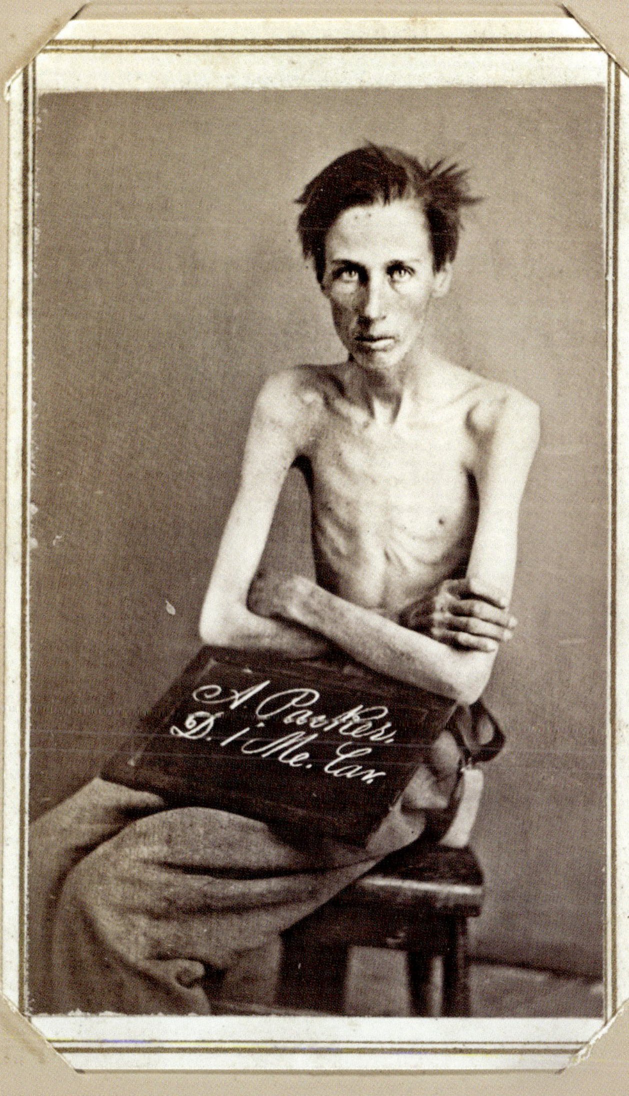

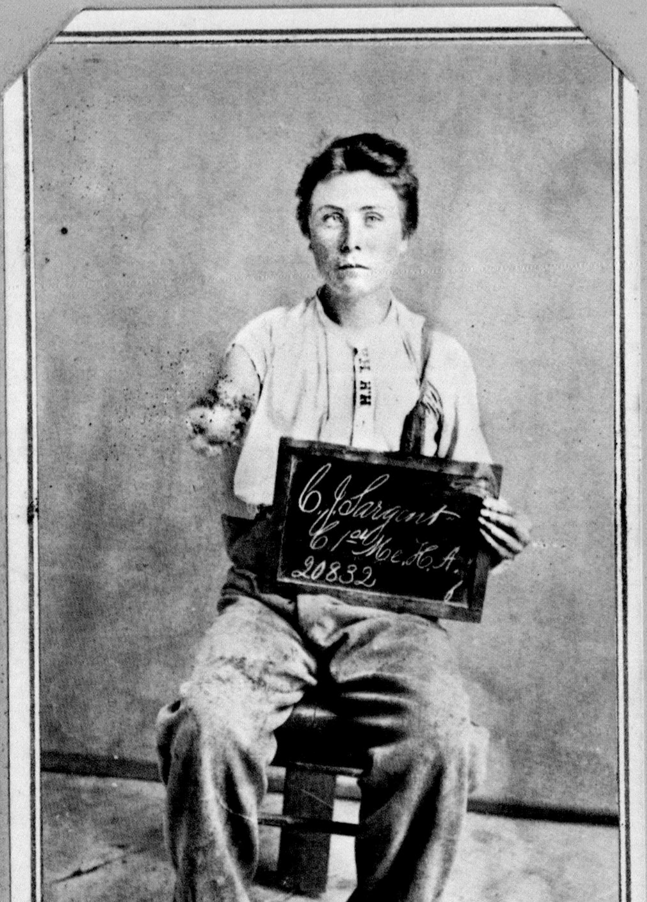

C.J. SARGENT
CO C 1 ME HA

PETERSBURG
APRIL 6, 1865

GSW RIGHT ELBOW.
AMPUTATION OF RIGHT ARM,
LOWER THIRD, BILATERAL FLAPS.
ON THE FIELD.

DISCHARGED JUNE 6, 1865

F.C. FOSS
4 ME BAT

PETERSBURG
MARCH 8, 1865

GSW RIGHT KNEE.

DISCHARGED JUNE 24, 1865

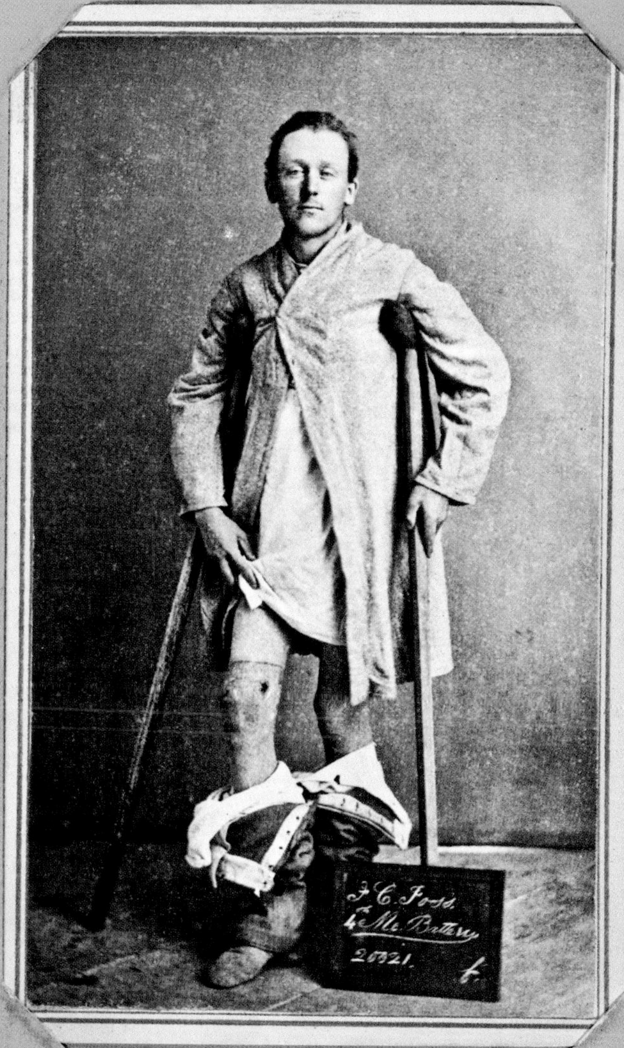

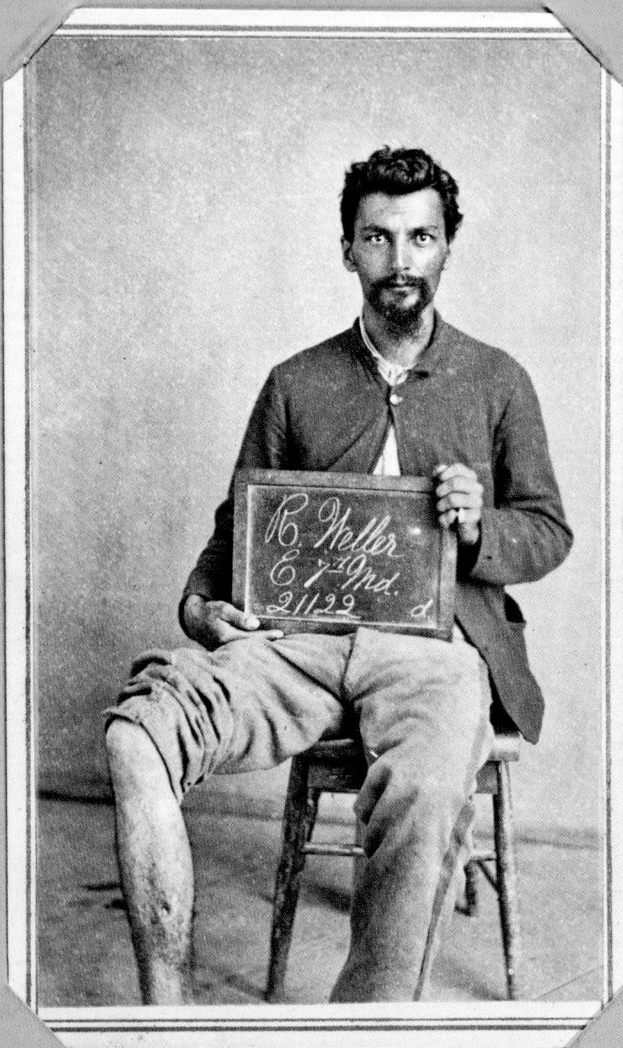

MARYLAND

R. WELLER
CO E 7 MD

APPOMATTOX COURT HOUSE
(THE DAY LEE SURRENDERED)
APRIL 9, 1865

GSW, LEFT LEG.

DISCHARGED JUNE 2, 1865

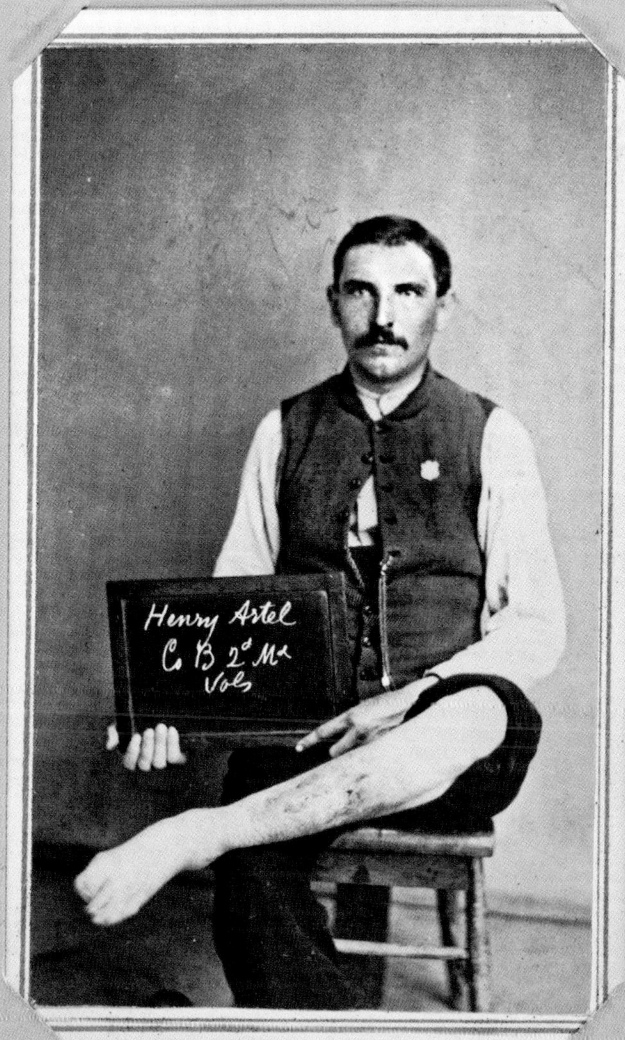

HENRY ARTEL
CO B 2 MD

PETERSBURG
APRIL 2, 1865

GSW, LEFT LEG.

DISCHARGED SEP 6, 1865

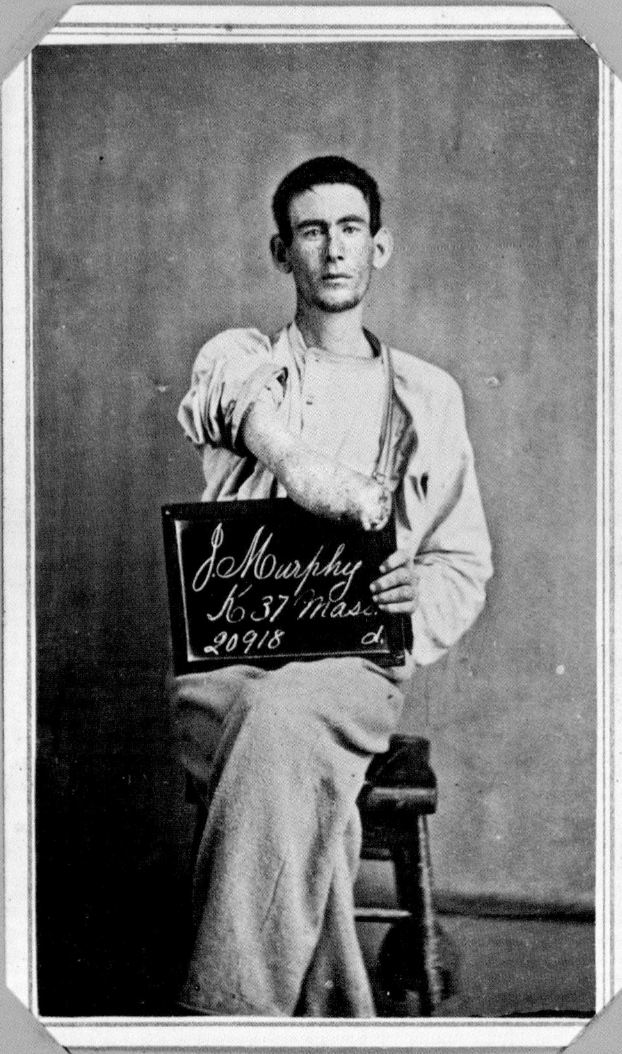

MASSACHUSETTS

J. MURPHY
CO K 37 MASS

SAYLER'S CREEK
(HARPER'S FARM)
APRIL 6, 1865

AMPUTATION OF RIGHT FOREARM, MIDDLE THIRD BY CIRCULAR METHOD. ON THE FIELD.

DISCHARGED JULY 10, 1865

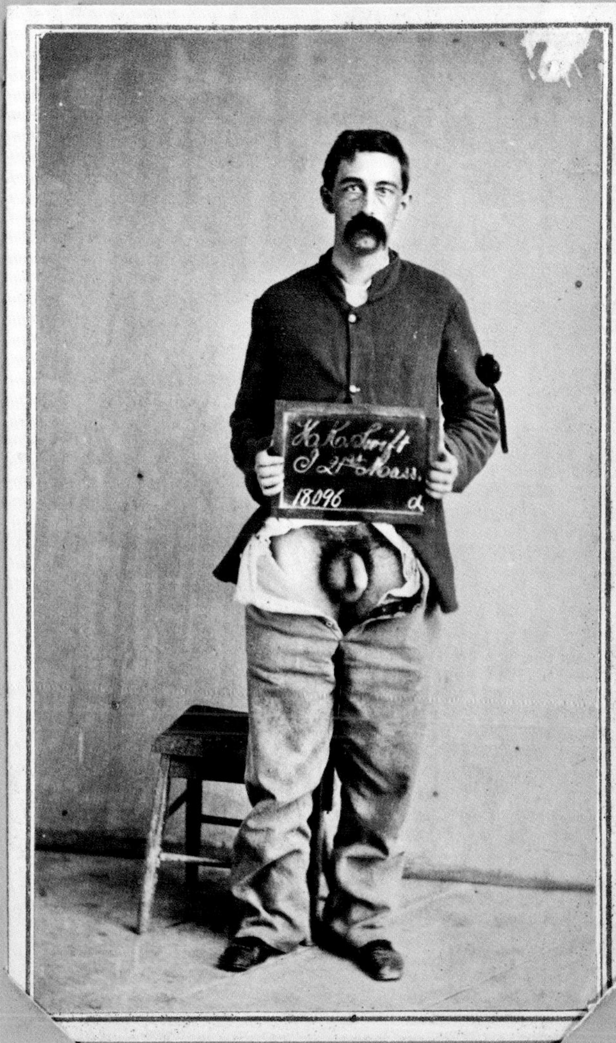

H.K. SWIFT

21 MASS

SCROTAL HERNIA.

DISCHARGED MAY 30, 1865

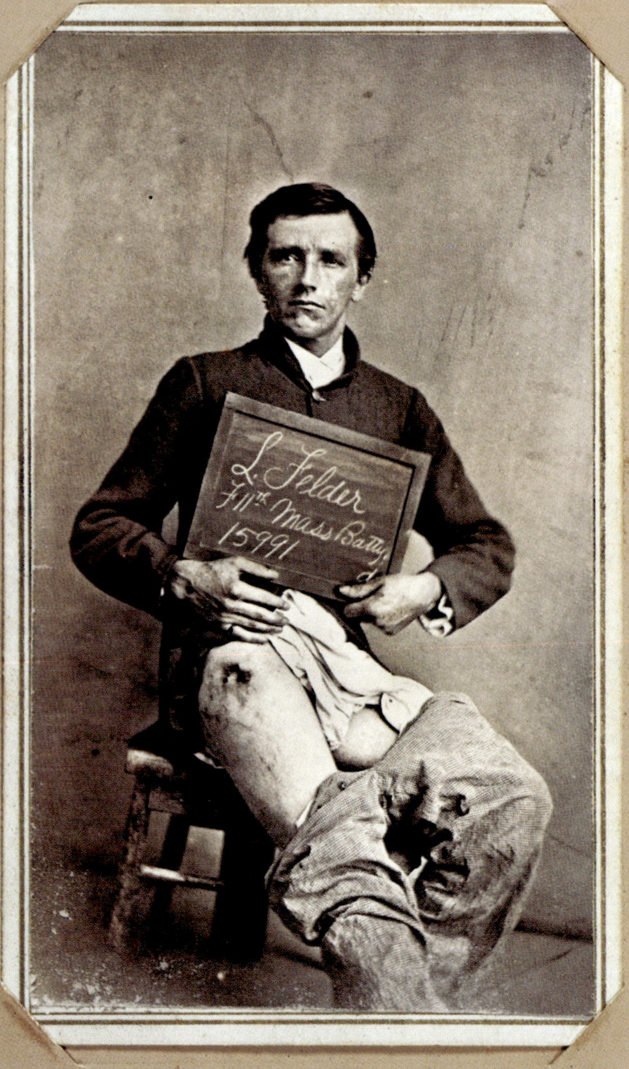

L. FELDER
CO F 11 MASS BAT

PETERSBURG
JUNE 16, 1864

GSW RIGHT THIGH &
FRONT FOREARM.

DISCHARGED JULY 18, 1865

N.E. HOWLAND
CO E 58 MASS

PETERSBURG
JUNE 6, 1864

GSW, LEFT LEG.

DISCHARGED MAY 31, 1865

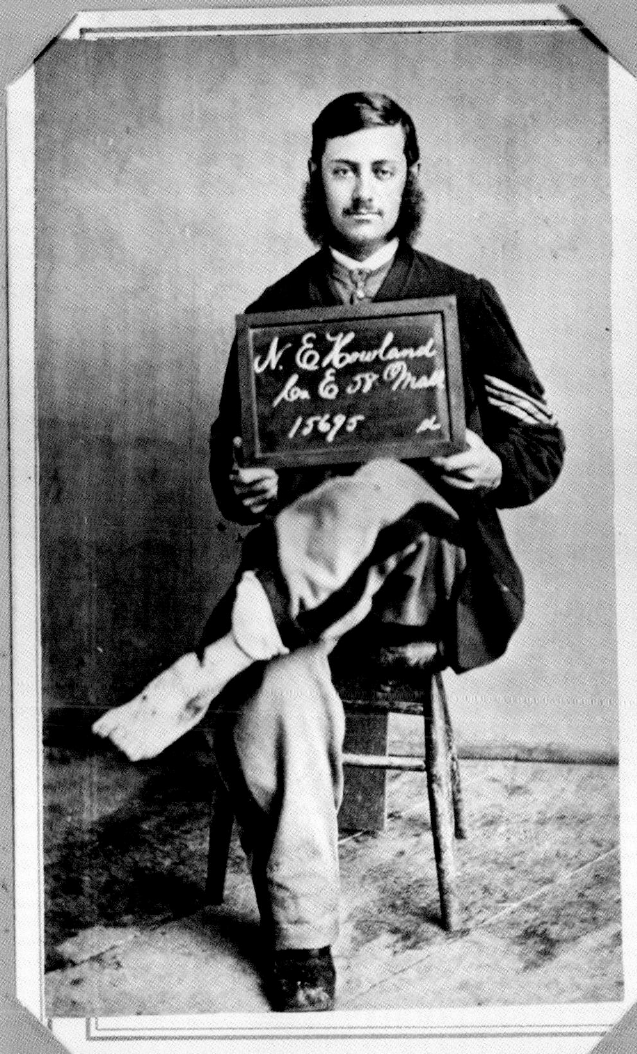

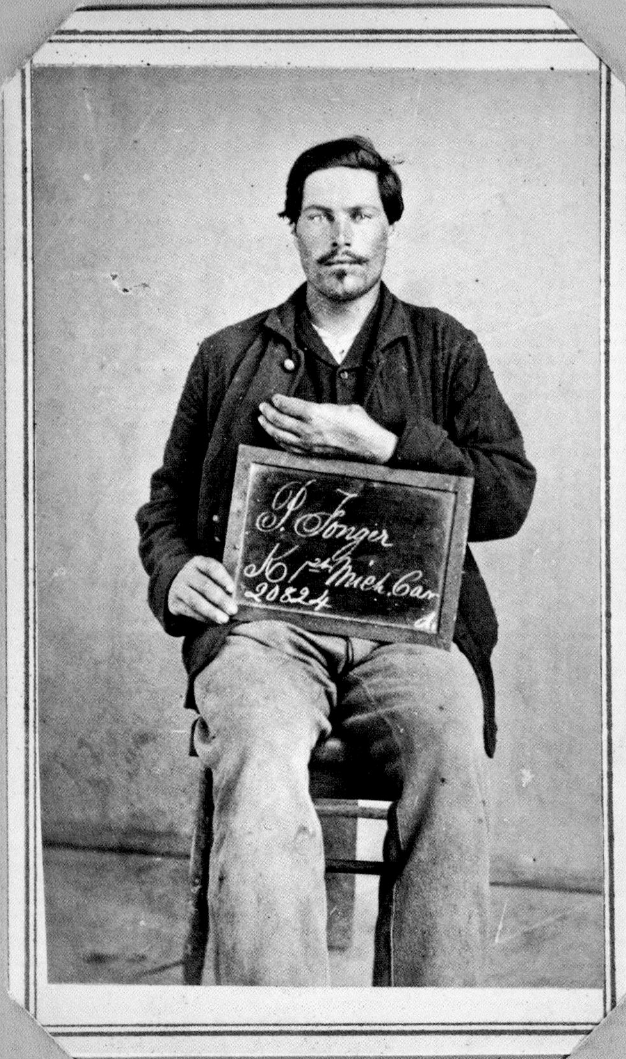

MICHIGAN

P. FONGER
CO K 1 MICH CAV

PETERSBURG
APRIL 6, 1865

GSW, THUMB OF LEFT HAND.
AMPUTATION OF THUMB.

DISCHARGED JUNE 28, 1865

S. BOYCE
CO B 5 MICH

WILDERNESS
MAY 6, 1864

GSW, FRACTURING
RIGHT THIGH.

DISCHARGED JUNE 14, 1865

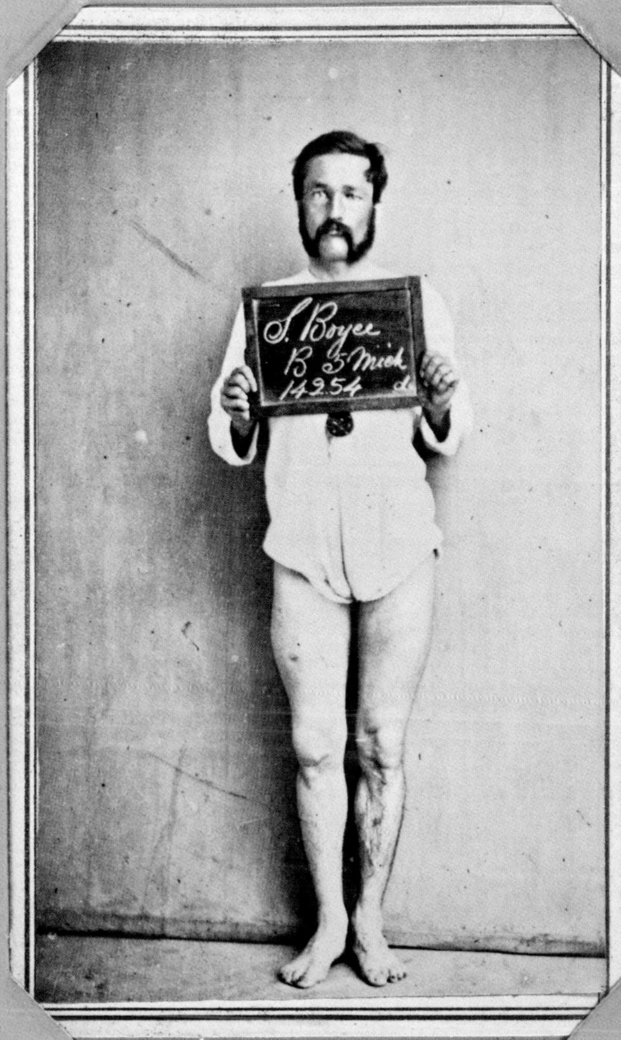

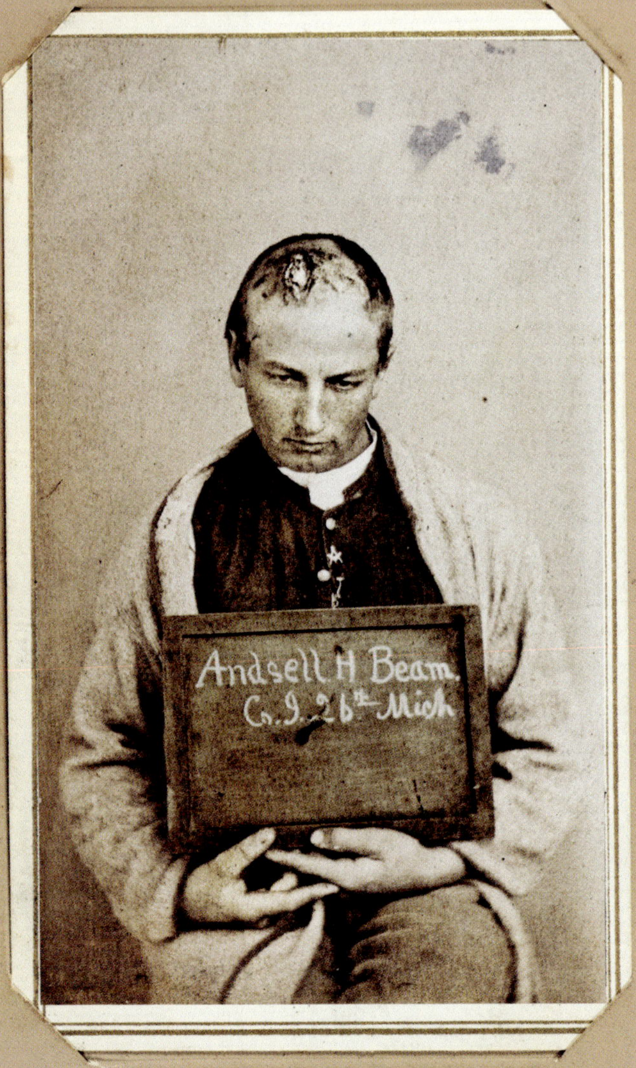

Aged 24, was admitted to HH, April 16th, 1865, with gunshot wound of head, injuring skull, upper anterior aspect. Wounded April 6th, 1865, at battle of Farmersville, Virginia. Progress favorable. Transferred to U.S.A. Gen. Hospital, Philadelphia, PA, May 18th, 1865. Doing well.

ANDSELL H. BEAM
CO J 26 MICH

FARMERSVILLE
APRIL 6, 1865

SABER WOUND ON HEAD.

TRANSFERRED MAY 18, 1865:
USA GEN HOSPITAL,
PHILADELPHIA

J.L. SECORD

CO H 5 MICH CAV

SOUTH SIDE RAILROAD
(PINES CHURCH)
APRIL 6, 1865

GSW, RIGHT HAND FINGER. AMPUTATION OF THE LITTLE FINGER ON THE FIELD.

DISCHARGED JUNE 29, 1865

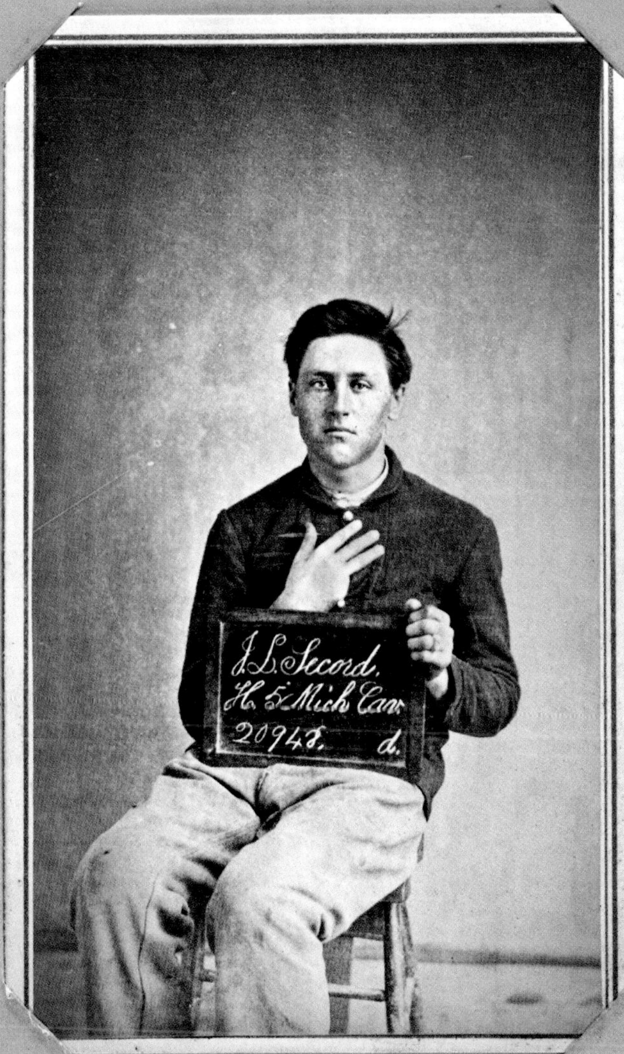

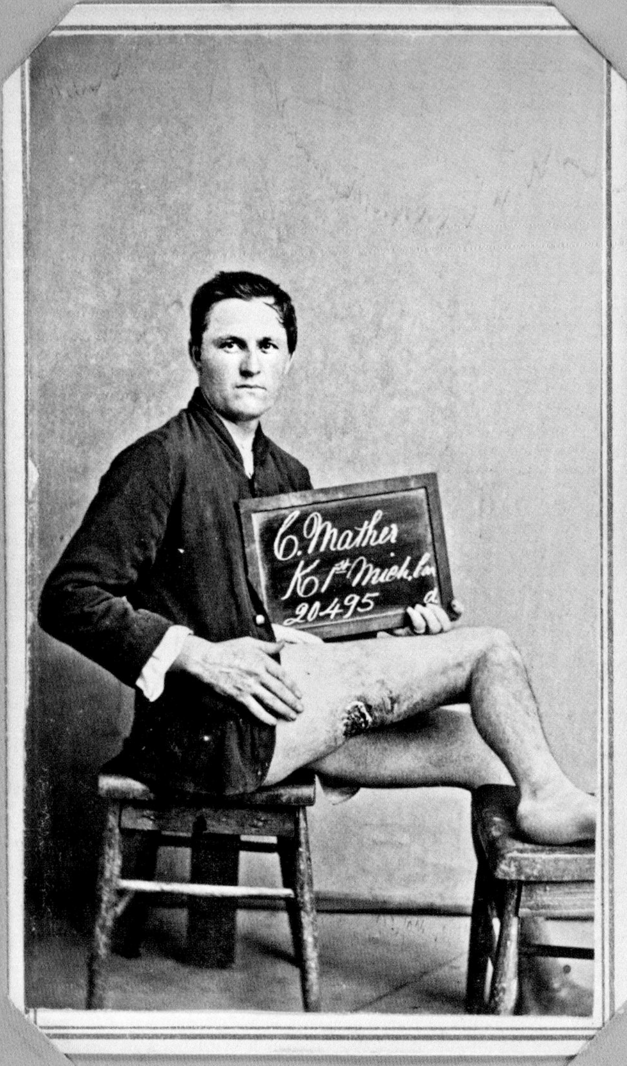

C. MATHER
CO K 1 MICH CAV

HATCHERS RUN
APRIL 1, 1865

GSW, RIGHT THIGH
THROUGH FASCIA & MUSCLES.

TRANSFERRED JULY 20, 1865:
LINCOLN USA GEN HOSPITAL

NEW HAMPSHIRE

S. EMERY
CO B 5 NH

COLD HARBOR
JUNE 3, 1864

GSW, LEFT FOREARM.

DISCHARGED JUNE 22, 1865

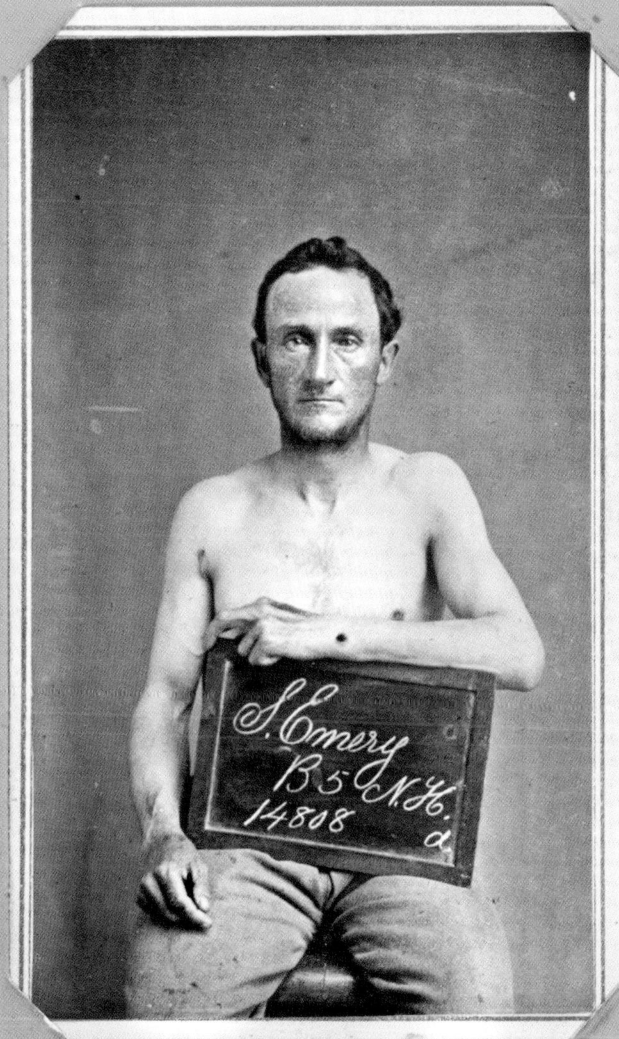

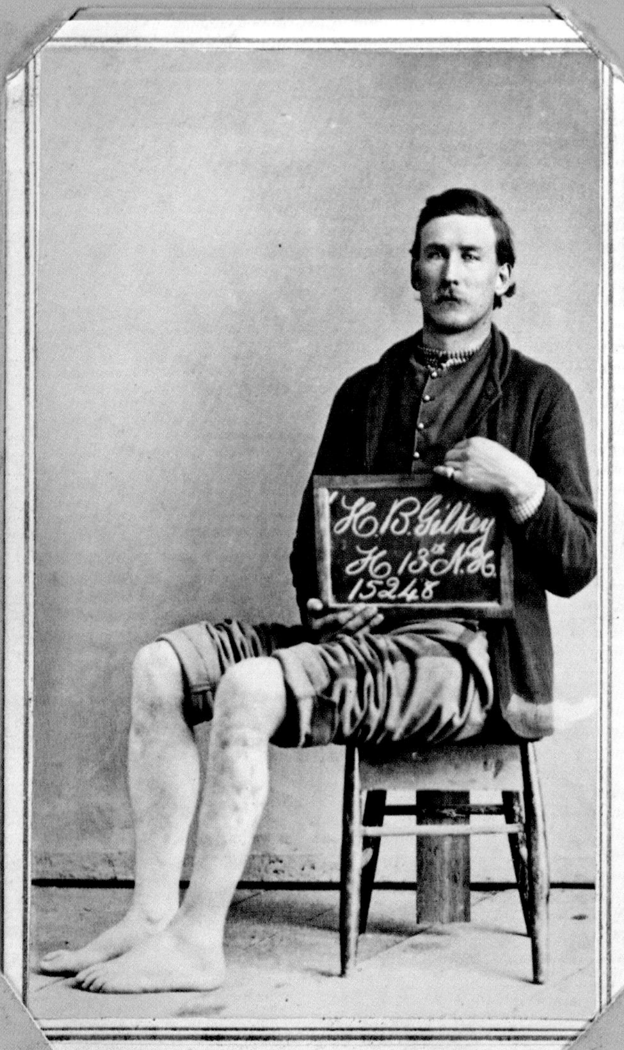

H.B. GILKEY
CO H 13 NH

COLD HARBOR
JUNE 1, 1864

GSW, LEFT LEG.

DISCHARGED APRIL 11, 1865

JOHN FOLSOM
CO D, 6 NH

GSW, SCALP.

DISCHARGED JUNE 14, 1865

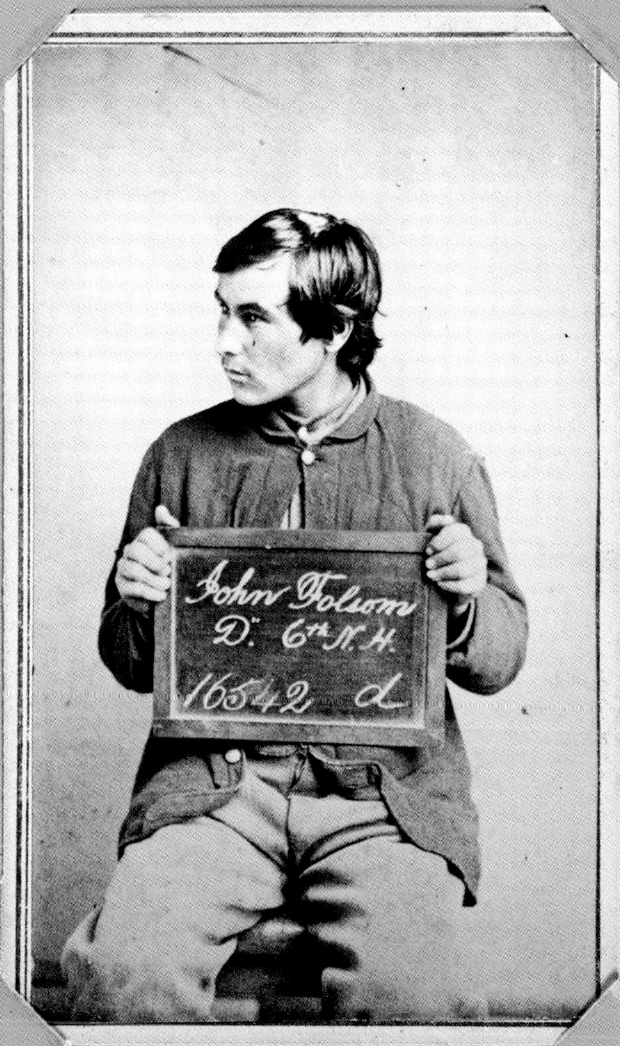

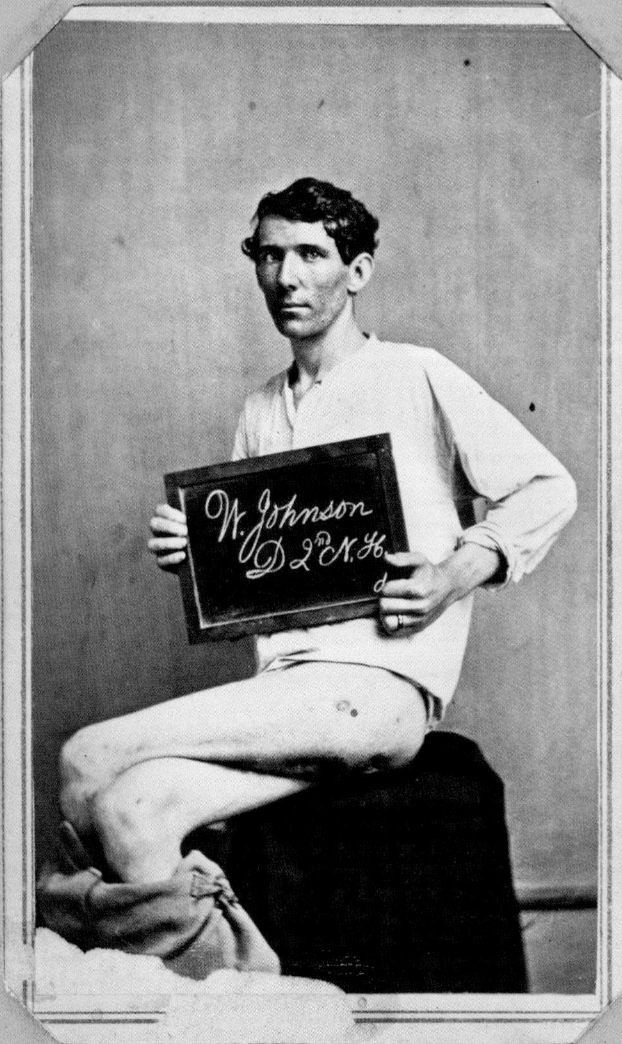

W. JOHNSON
CO D 2 NH

COLD HARBOR
JUNE 8, 1864

GSW, LEFT GLUTIAL MUSCLE.

DISCHARGED JULY 3, 1865

NEW JERSEY

E. KITCHELL
CO K 15 NJ

WORCHESTER
SEPTEMBER 19, 1864

GSW, LEFT ARM.

DISCHARGED JUNE 14, 1865

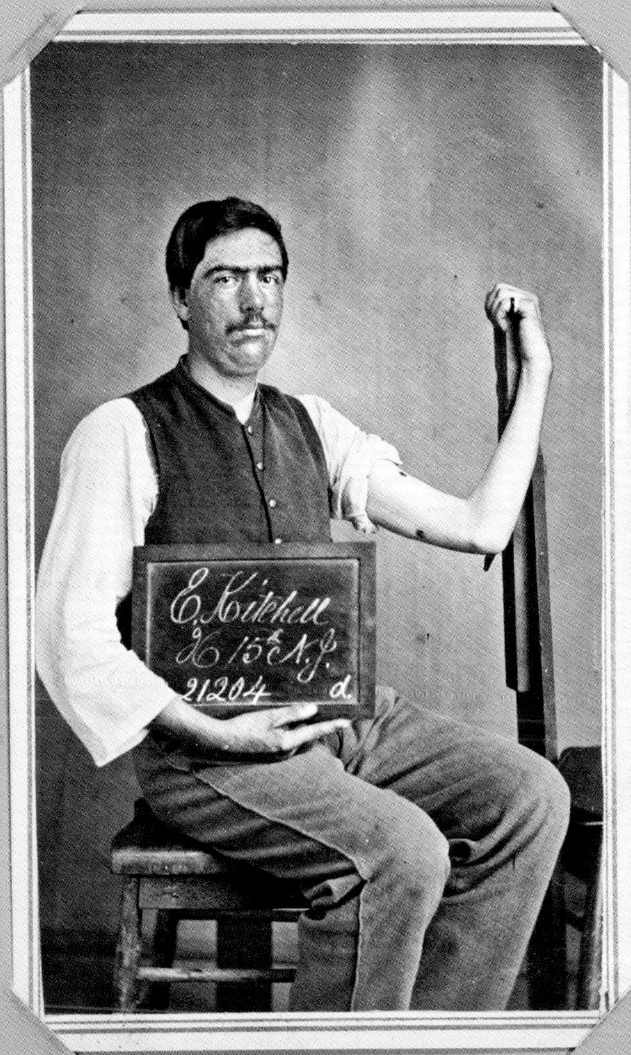

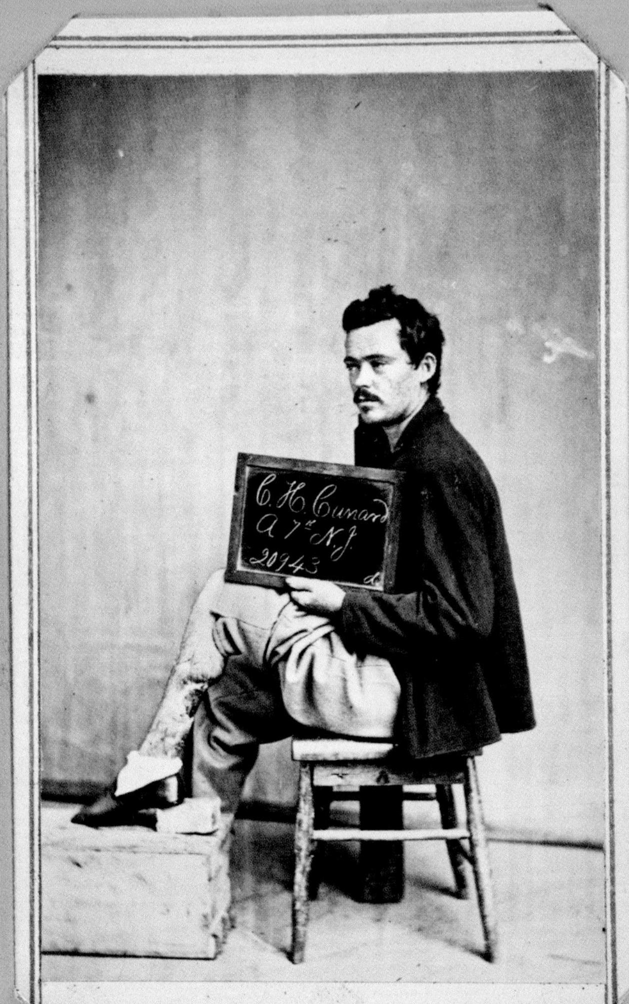

C.H. CUNARD
CO A 7 NJ

BATCHELOR'S HOME, VA
APRIL 7, 1865

GSW, LEFT LEG.

TRANSFERRED JULY 20, 1865:
LINCOLN USA GEN HOSPITAL

GILBERT HUNTER
CO A 1 NJ CAV

BURKES STATION
APRIL 6, 1865

GSW, LEFT ARM.

TRANSFERRED MAY 2, 1865:
USA GEN HOSPITAL, NEWARK

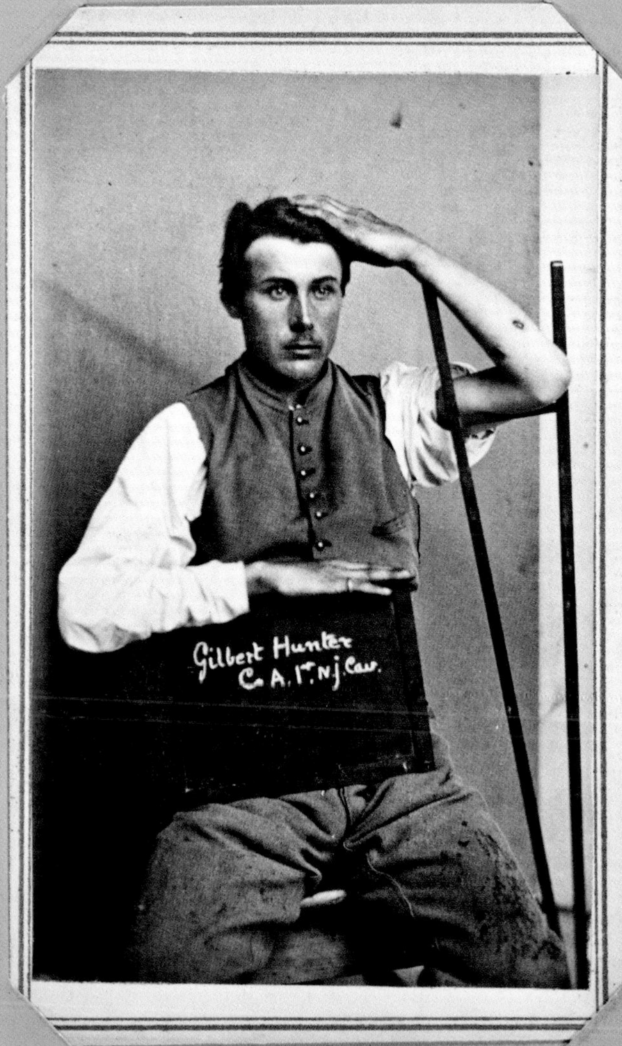

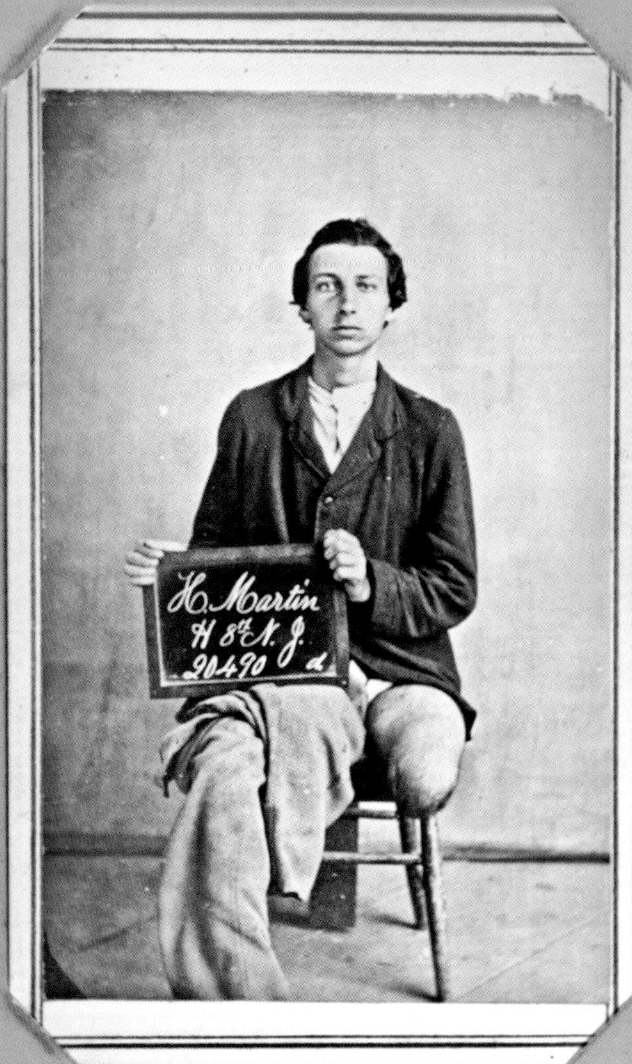

H. MARTIN

CO H 8 NJ

PETERSBURG

MARCH 31, 1865

GSW, LEFT THIGH.

CIRCULAR AMPUTATION,

ON FIELD.

TRANSFERRED JULY 1, 1865:

USA GEN HOSPITAL, DOUGLAS

NEW YORK

SGT. H. H. BROWER
CO C 10 NY ZOUAVE

SPOTSYLVANIA
MAY 10, 1864

GSW, RIGHT LEG.
AMPUTATION OF LEG.

DISCHARGED NOV 14, 1865

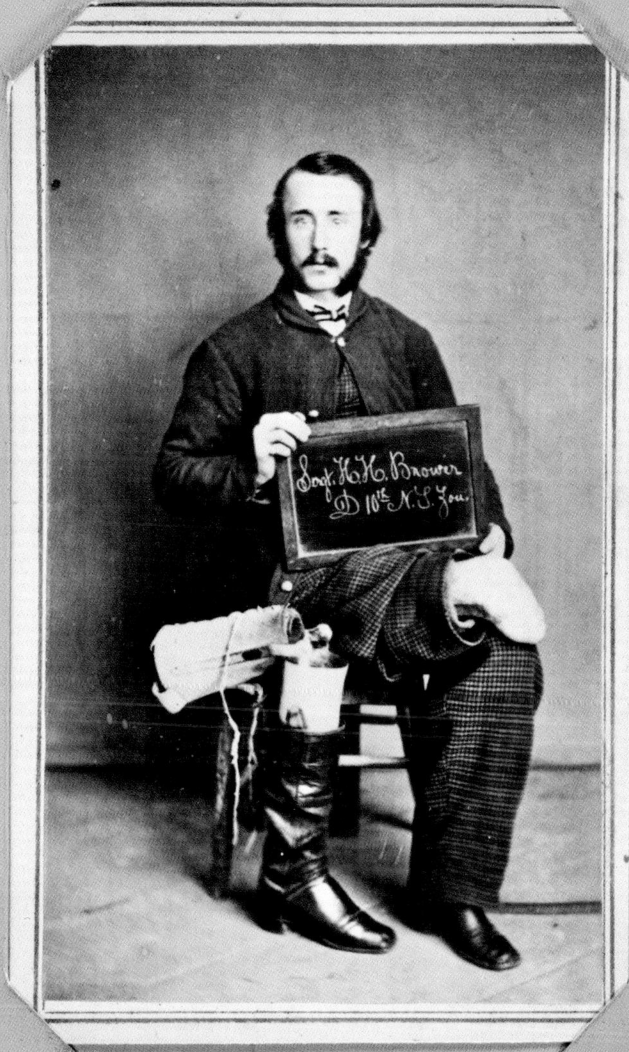

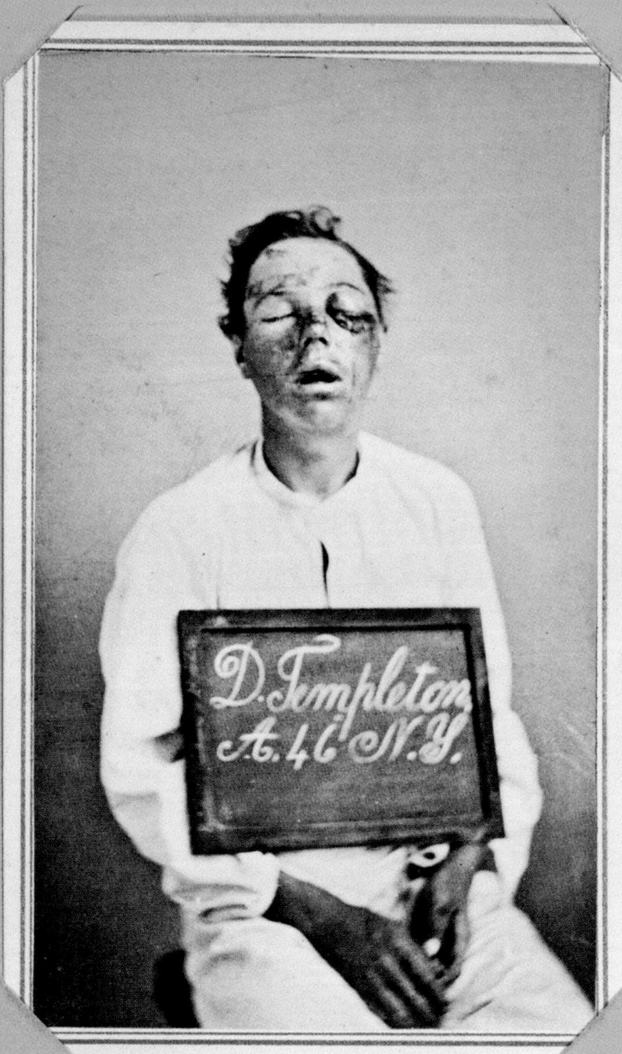

Age 16, was admitted to HH, April 5th 1865, with gunshot wound of the head. Ball hit left temple, just back of outer angle of eye, grazing malar bone and eyeball, destroying sight; passed off producing flesh wound of the tip of the nose. Was wounded at Petersburg April 2nd 1865. He is now well, June 1st, 1865.

DAVID R. TEMPLETON

CO A 46 NY

PETERSBURG

APRIL 2, 1865

GSW, LEFT EYE.

AT TIME OF ADMISSION.

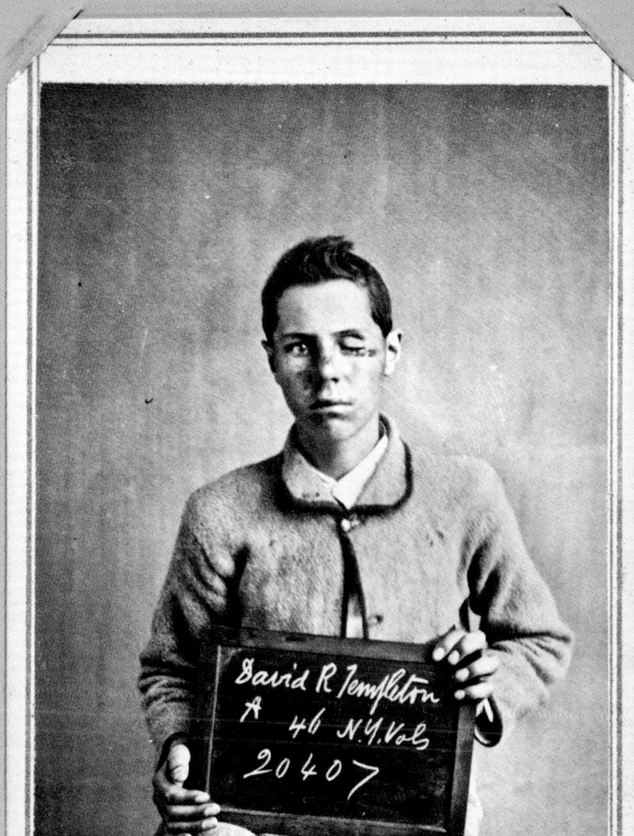

GSW, LEFT EYE.
AT TIME OF DISCHARGE.

DISCHARGED MAY 30, 1865

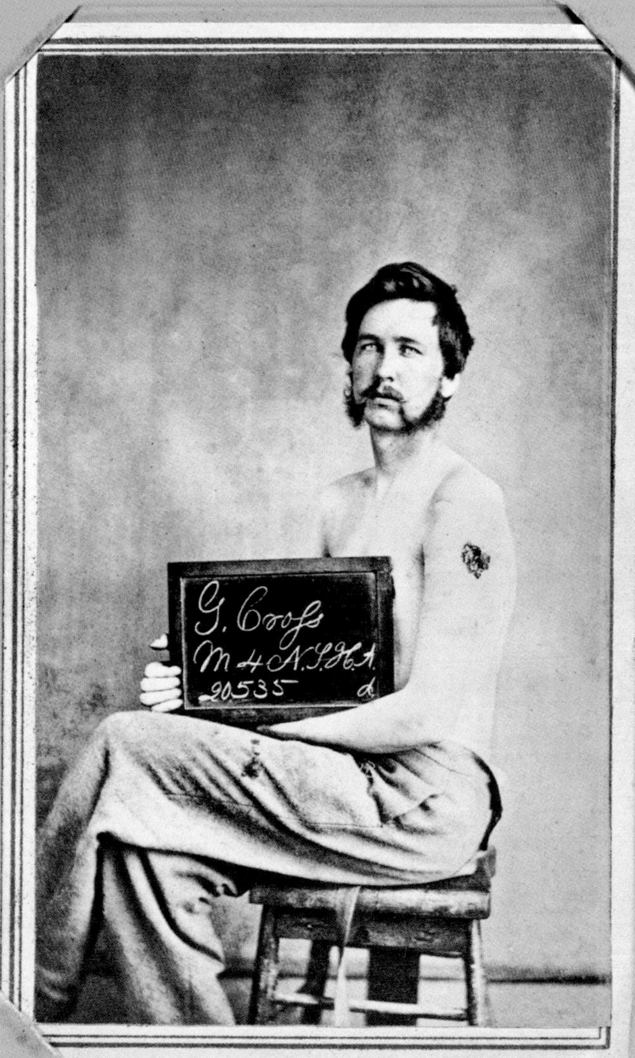

G. CROSS

CO M 4 NY HA

PETERSBURG

(VAUGHN ROAD)

APRIL 2, 1865

GSW, LEFT ARM, UPPER THIRD.

DISCHARGED JULY 24, 1865

H.L. LANNING
CO C 86 NY

WILDERNESS
MAY 11, 1864

GSW, LEFT GROIN.

DISCHARGED MAY 30, 1865

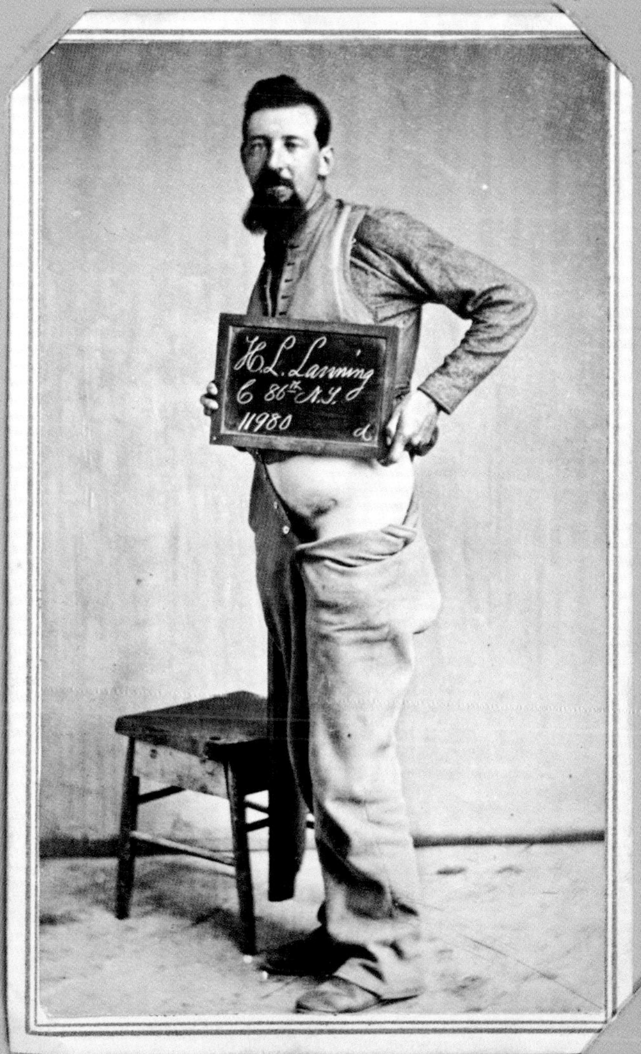

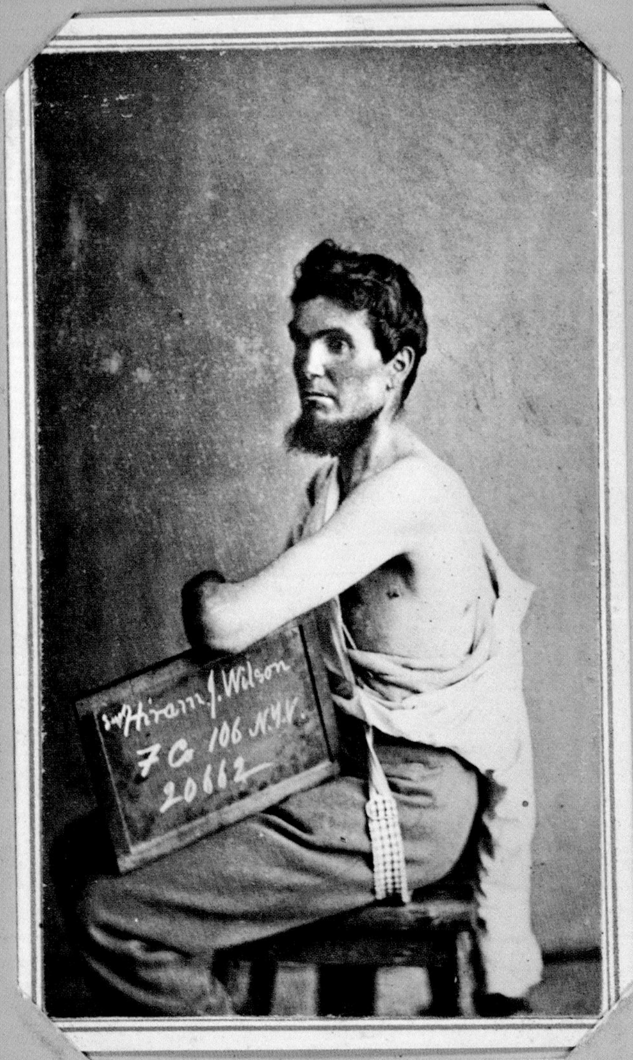

SGT. HIRAM J. WILSON
CO F 106 NY

PETERSBURG
APRIL 2, 1865

GSW, LEFT SIDE.

DISCHARGED MAY 27, 1865

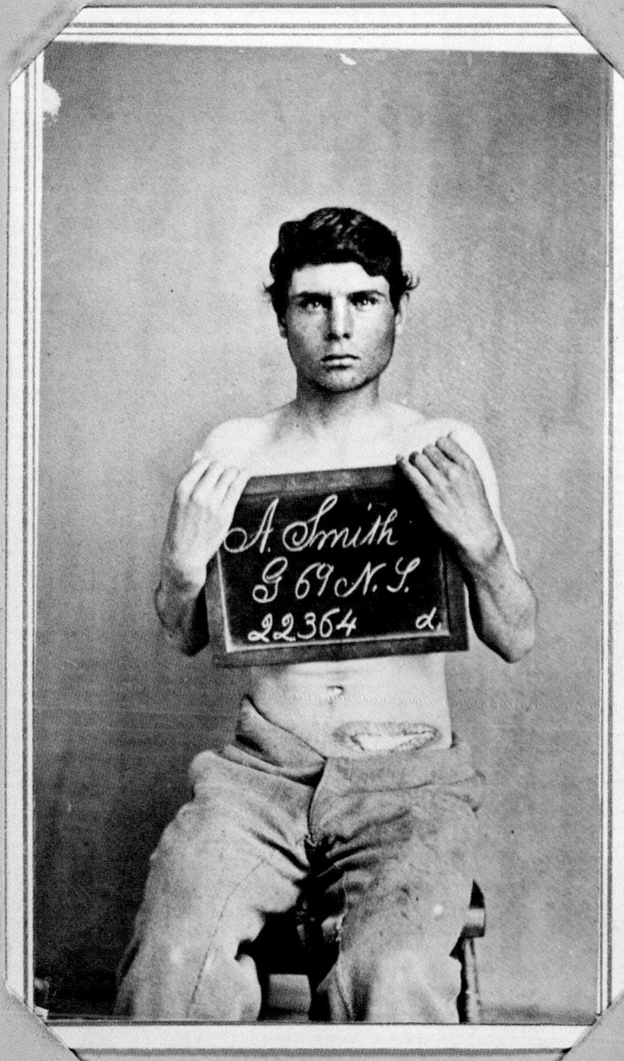

A. SMITH

CO G 69 NY

SOUTHSIDE RAIL ROAD

JUNE 16, 1864

GSW, EXTENSION OF
CICATRIX OF ABDOMEN.

DISCHARGED JULY 27, 1864

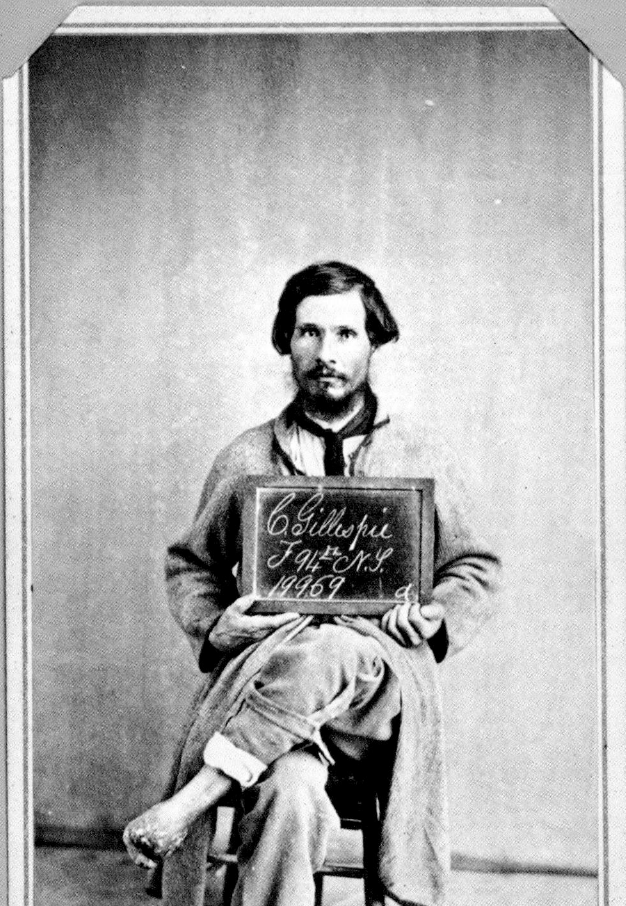

C. GILLESPIE

CO F 94 NY

PETERSBURG

MARCH 19, 1865

ACCIDENTAL GSW,
LEFT FOOT AMPUTATION.
"CHARTRAND METHOD"
ON THE FIELD.

DISCHARGED MAY 29, 1865

D.A. ROBINSON
CO B 151 NY

RIGHT INGUINAL HERNIA.

DISCHARGED JULY 12, 1865

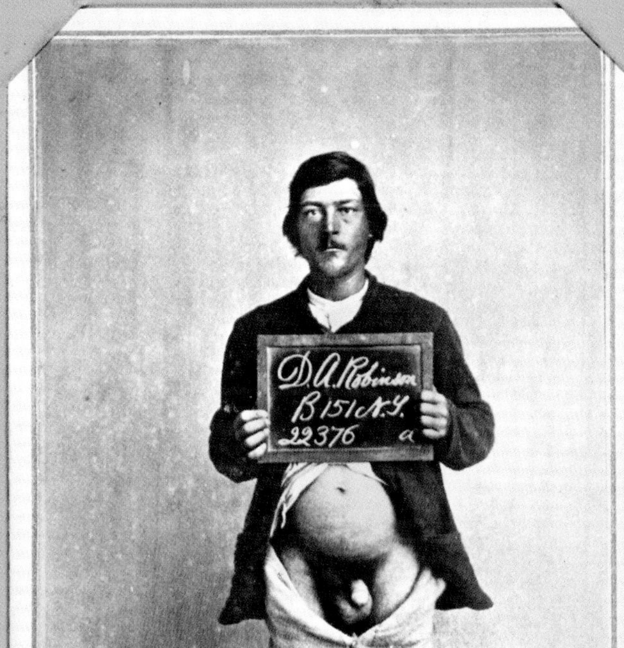

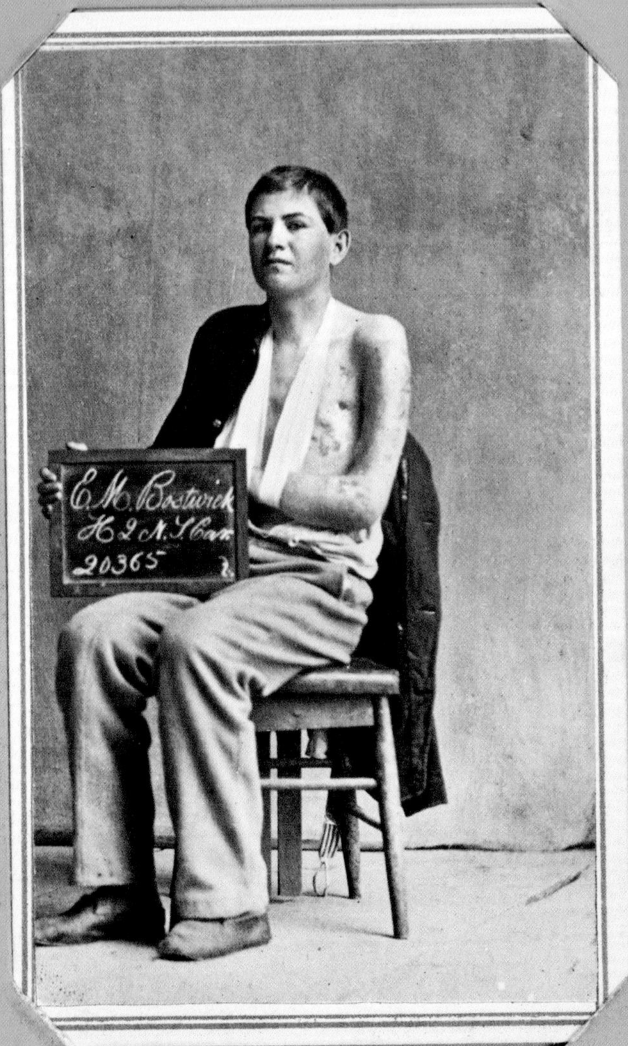

E.M. BOSTWICK

CO H 2 NY CAV

PETERSBURG

APRIL 1, 1865

GSW, LEFT ARM.
RESECTION OF LEFT HUMERUS
MIDDLE THIRD. THREE INCHES
OF BONE REMOVED.

TRANSFERRED JUNE 13, 1865:
USA HOSPITAL, ROCHESTER, NY

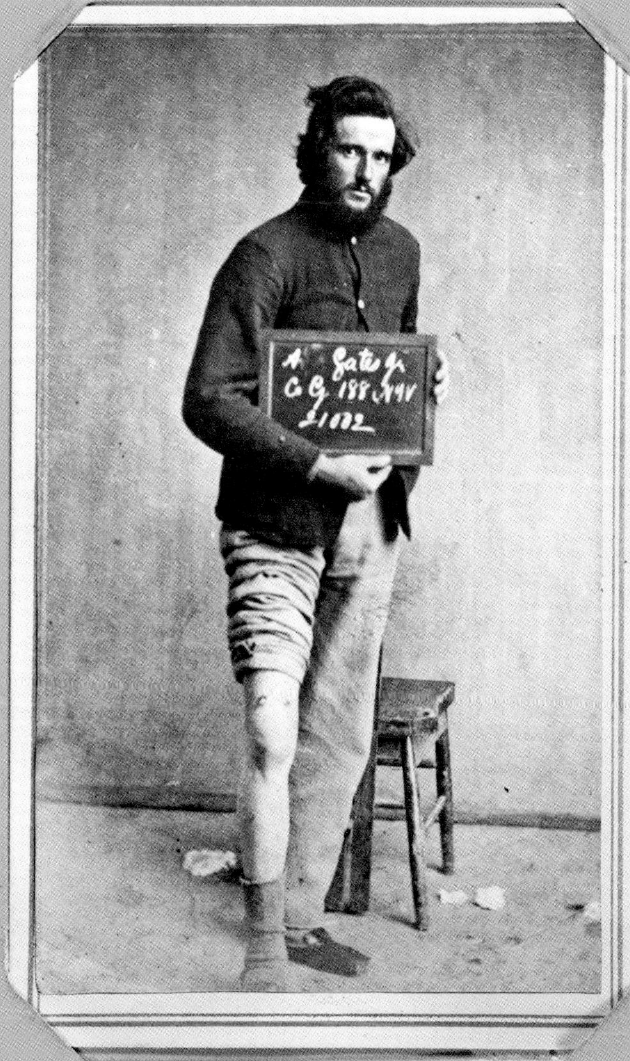

A. GATES JR.
CO G 188 NY

SUTHERLAND
APRIL 1, 1865

GSW, GROIN & RIGHT THIGH.

DISCHARGED MAY 29, 1865

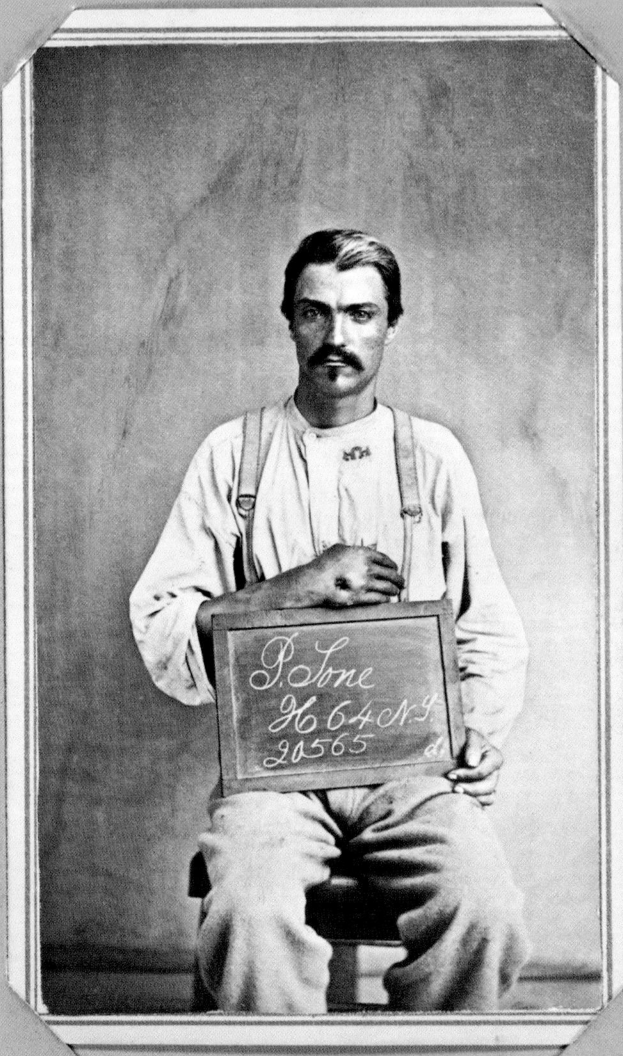

P. LONE
CO H 64 NY

SOUTH SIDE RAIL ROAD
MARCH 31, 1865

GSW, RIGHT HAND.

DISCHARGED JULY 12, 1865

MICHAEL ASHEN
CO H 9 NY CAV

TYPHOID FEVER.

DISCHARGED SEP 28, 1865

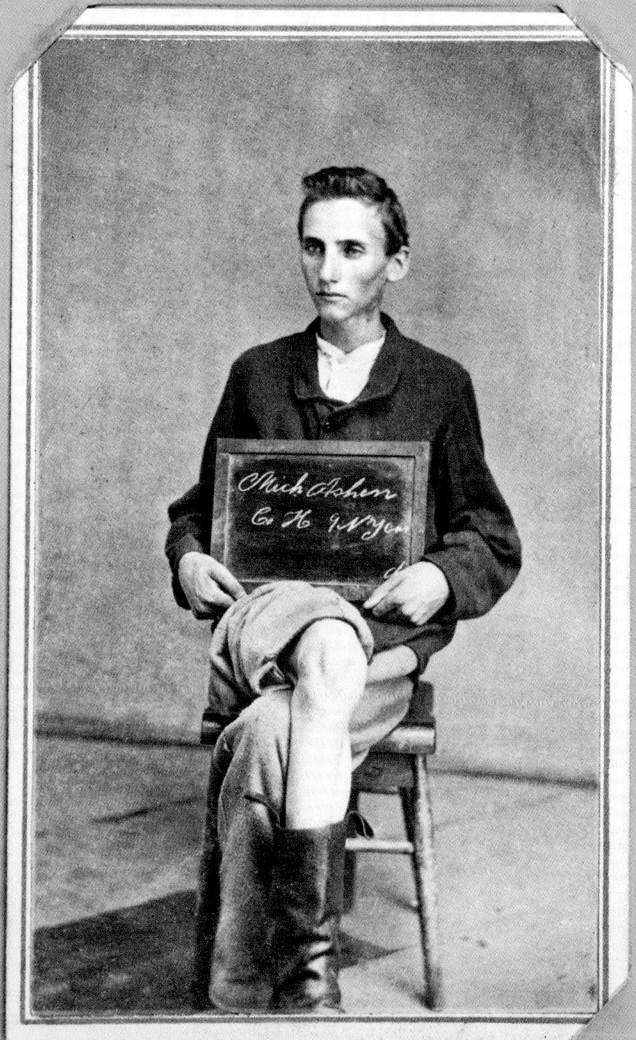

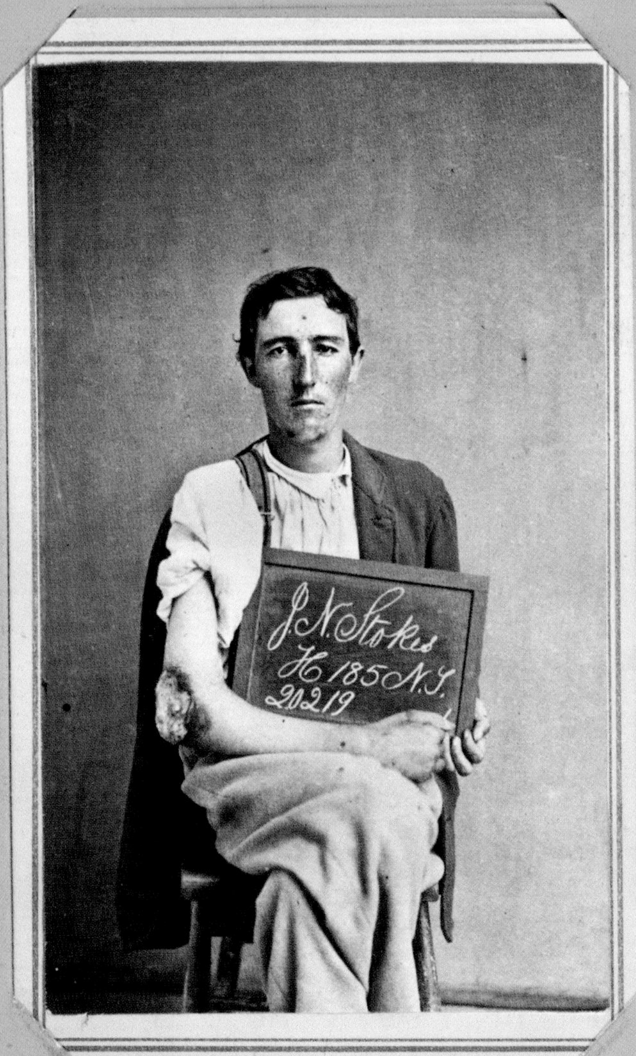

J.N. STOKES
CO H 185 NY

GRAVELLY RUN
MARCH 29, 1865

GSW, FRONT RIGHT FOREARM, FRACTURING INNER CONDYLE OF HUMERUS.

DISCHARGED JULY 5, 1865

Admitted to HH, May 7th, 1865, convalescent from GSW of left hip and abdomen. Wounded by minie ball before Petersburg, VA. June 18, 1864. The ball entered the umbilical region of abdomen, making its exit from left lumbar region fracturing crest of left ilium in its course. The exit of wound was followed by gangrene causing contraction and adhesions of muscles to ilium. Discharged June 25th. Wounds entirely healed.

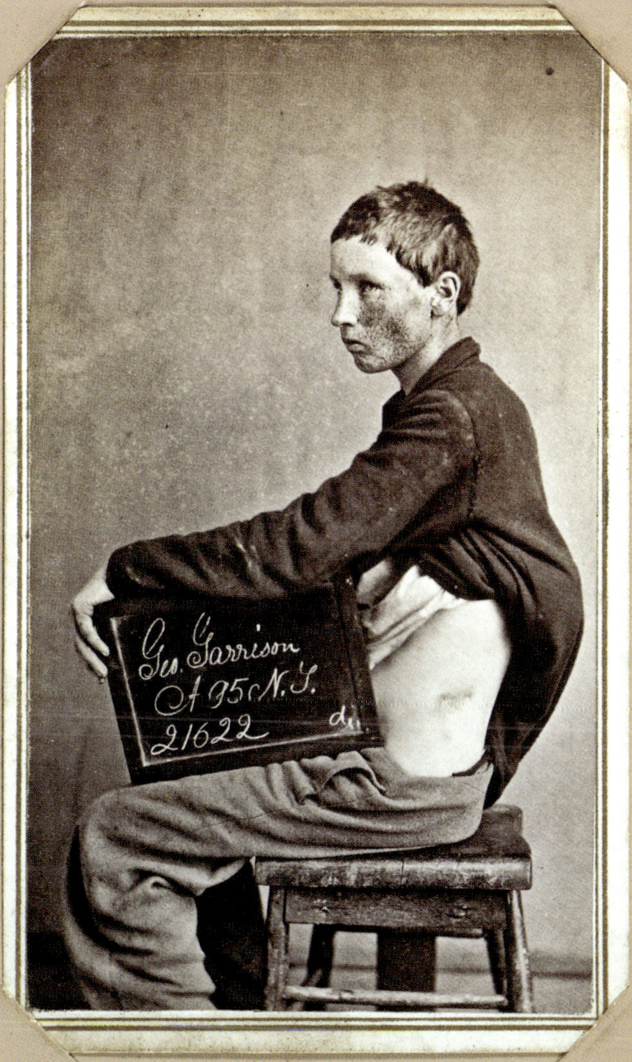

GEORGE GARRISON

CO A 95 NY

PETERSBURG

JUNE 18, 1864

GSW, HIP & ABDOMEN.

DISCHARGED JUNE 25, 1865

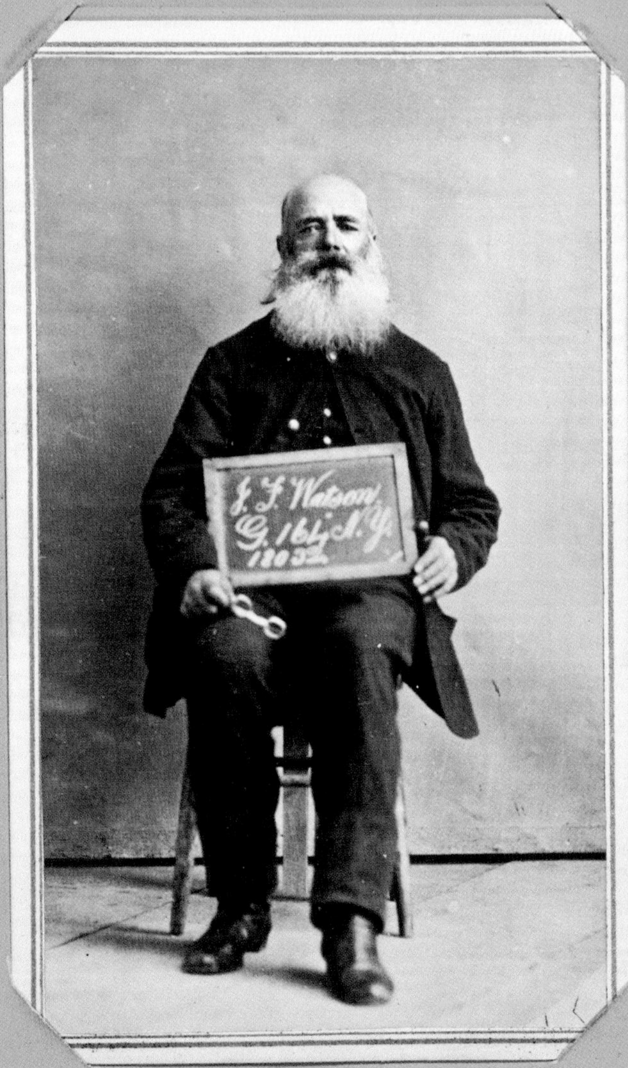

J.F. WATSON
CO G 164 NY

DEBILITY

DISCHARGED JUNE 12, 1865

Aged 18, admitted to HH, April 5, 1865, suffering from amputation of middle ring, little finger and metacarpal bones of same, result of gunshot wound, right hand; extent of injury unknown, apparently single flap from palmar surface; on field; operation and anesthetics unknown. Wounded at battle of Hatcher's Run, VA, March 25, 1865. On admission, the constitutional state of patient and condition of injured parts were good – parts granulating finely. Treatment, simple dressing; no unfavorable symptoms occurred, and parts healed kindly. Patient has good use of forefinger and thumb.

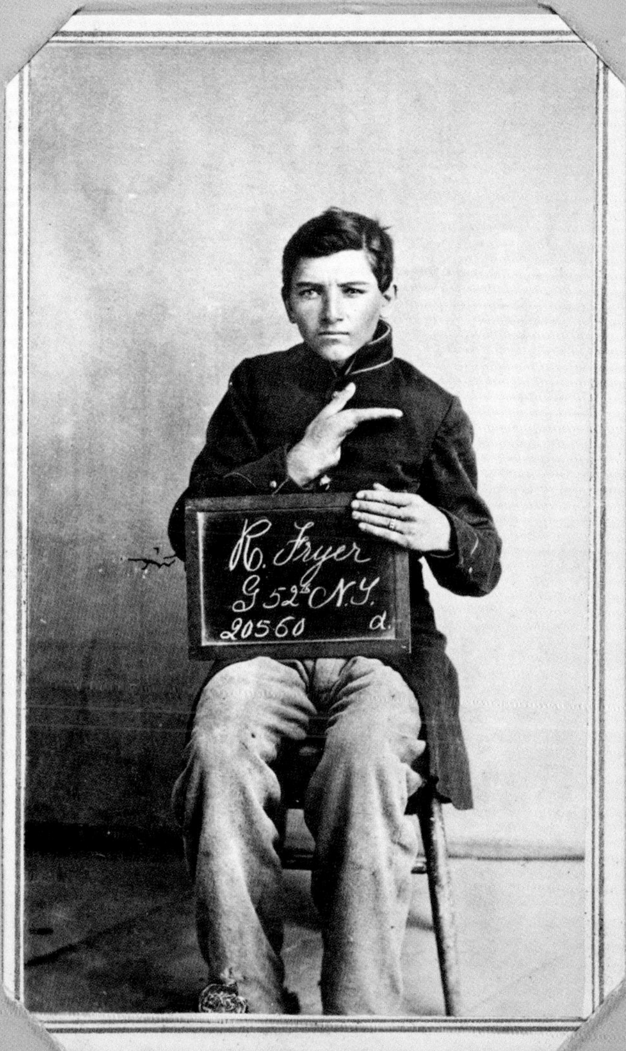

ROBERT FRYER
CO G 52 NY

HATCHER'S RUN
MARCH 25, 1865

GSW, RIGHT FINGERS.
AMPUTATION OF MIDDLE,
RING & LITTLE FINGER.

DISCHARGED JULY 28, 1865

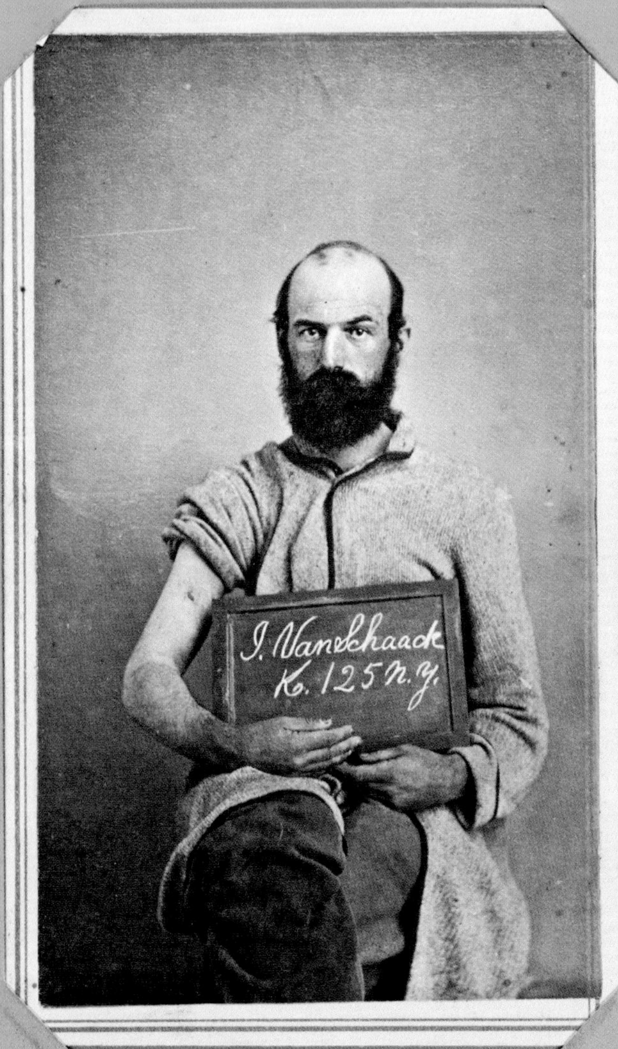

J. VAN SCHAACK
CO K 125 NY

HATCHER'S RUN
MARCH 31, 1865

GSW, RIGHT ARM.

TRANSFERRED MAY 12, 1865:
USA GEN HOSPITAL, TROY, NY

GEROME HOW
CO B 122 NY

SPOTTSYLVANIA
MAY 12, 1864

GSW, LEFT HAND.
AMPUTATION OF LEFT
INDEX FINGER.

DISCHARGED MAY 29, 1865

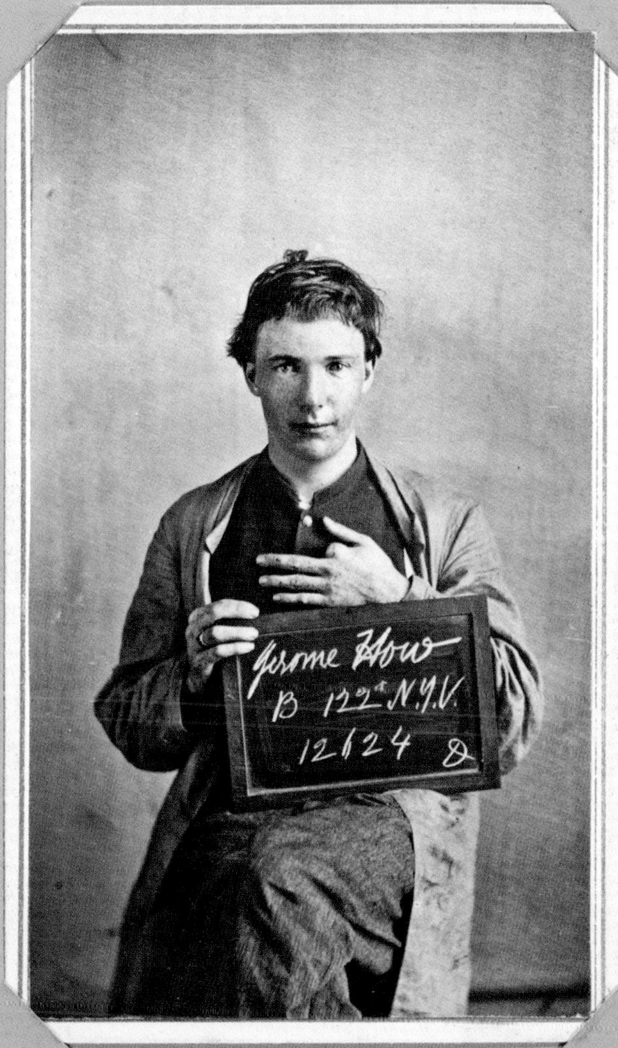

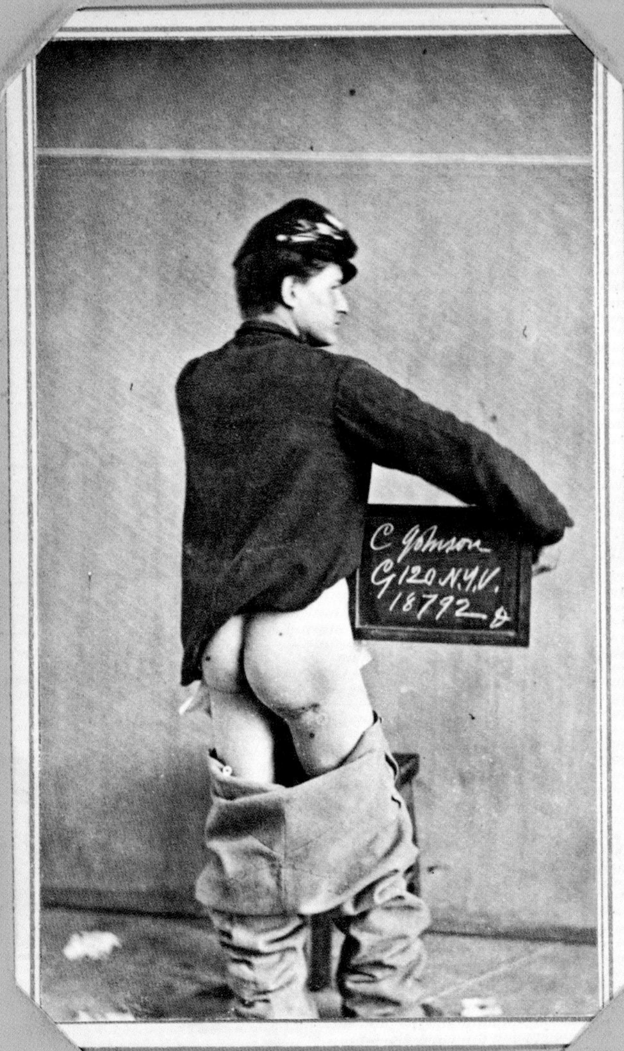

C. JOHNSON
CO G 120 NY

PETERSBURG,
NOVEMBER 6, 1864

GSW, RIGHT THIGH.

DISCHARGED MAY 29, 1865

B. REYNOLDS
CO C 154 NY

GANGRENE.

TRANSFERRED MAY 29, 1865:
USA GEN HOSPITAL,
PHILADELPHIA

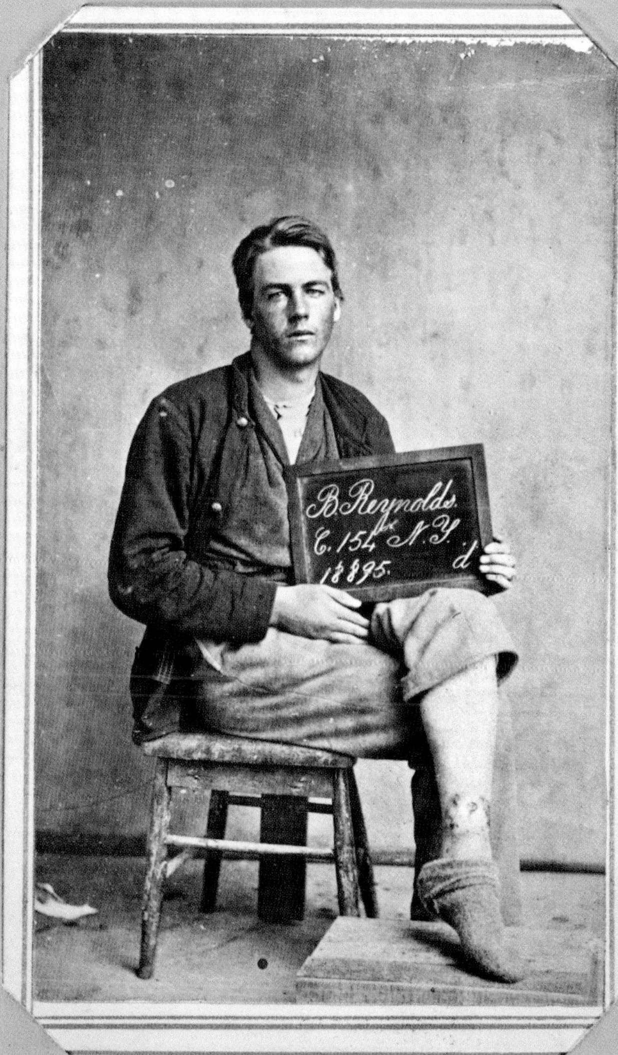

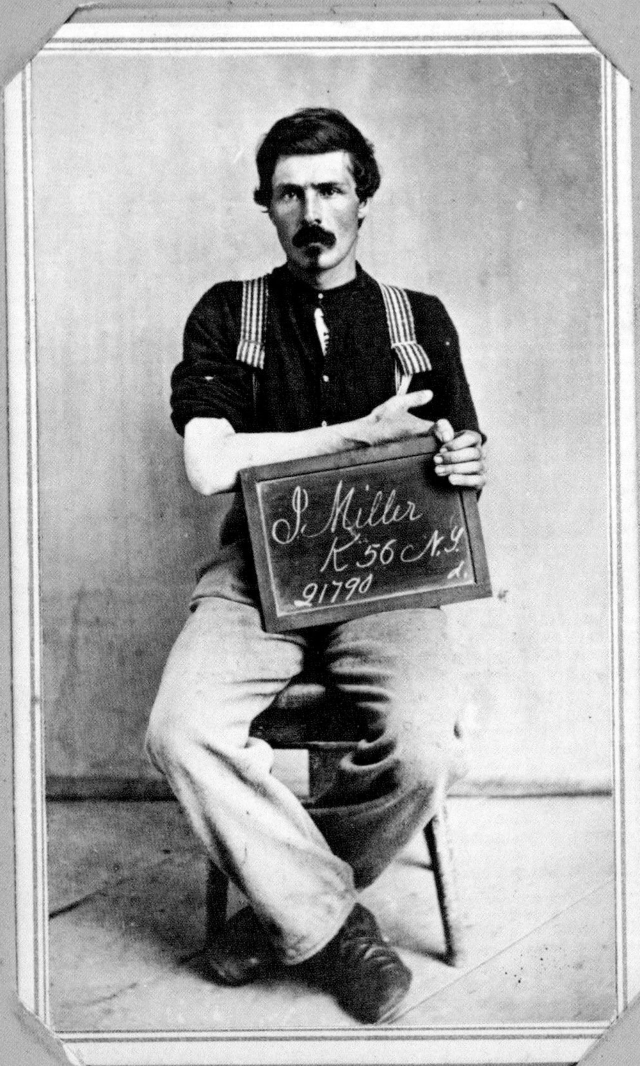

J. MILLER
CO K 56 NY

BANKSVILLE
APRIL 23, 1865

GSW, FRONT RIGHT ARM
FRACTURING HUMEROUS.

DISCHARGED JULY 10, 1865

F. CHURCH
CO D 1 NY CAV

PETERSBURG
APRIL 6, 1865

GSW, NECK.

DISCHARGED JUNE 21, 1865

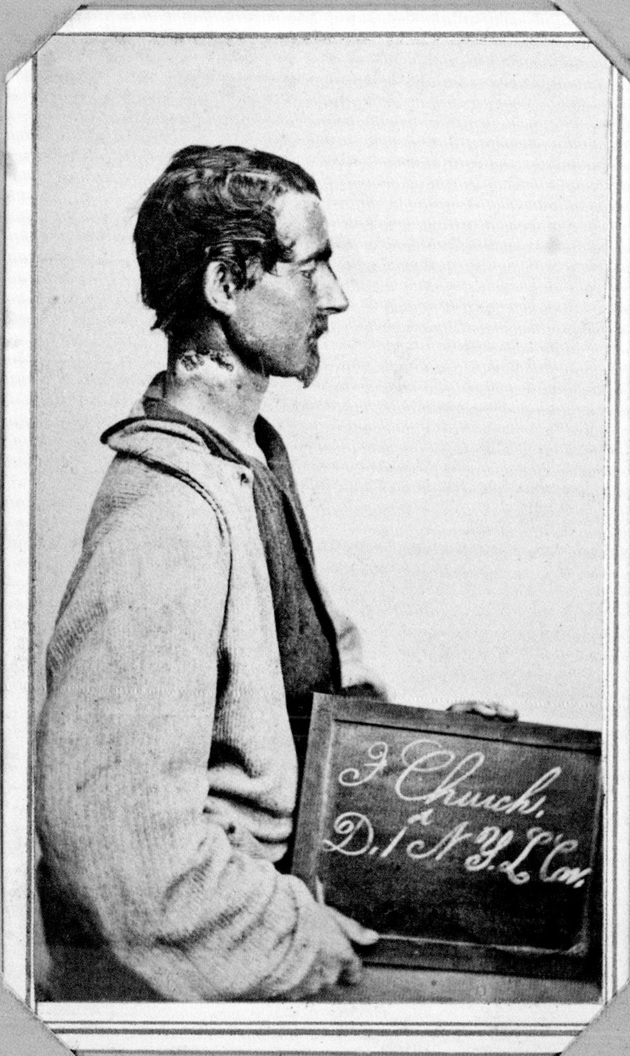

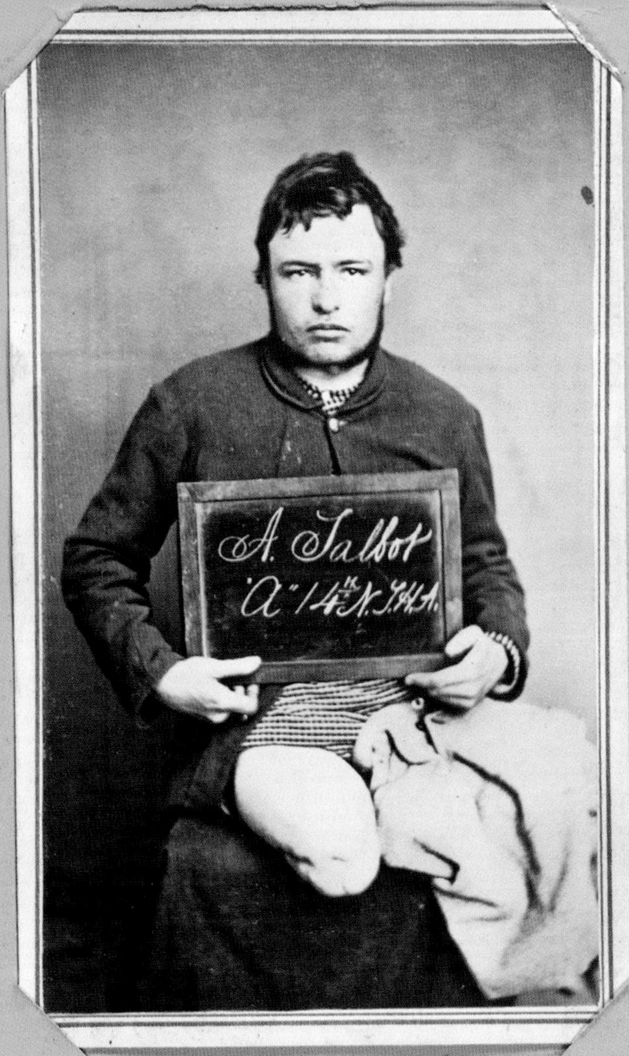

ANDRIE TALBOT

CO A 14 NY HA

PETERSBURG

MARCH 2, 1865

GSW, RIGHT THIGH.

AMPUTATION AT THIGH.

DISCHARGED NOV 28, 1865

J. KELLY
CO E 42 NY

WILDERNESS
MAY 6, 1864

GSW, LEFT SHOULDER.

DISCHARGED JUNE 22, 1865

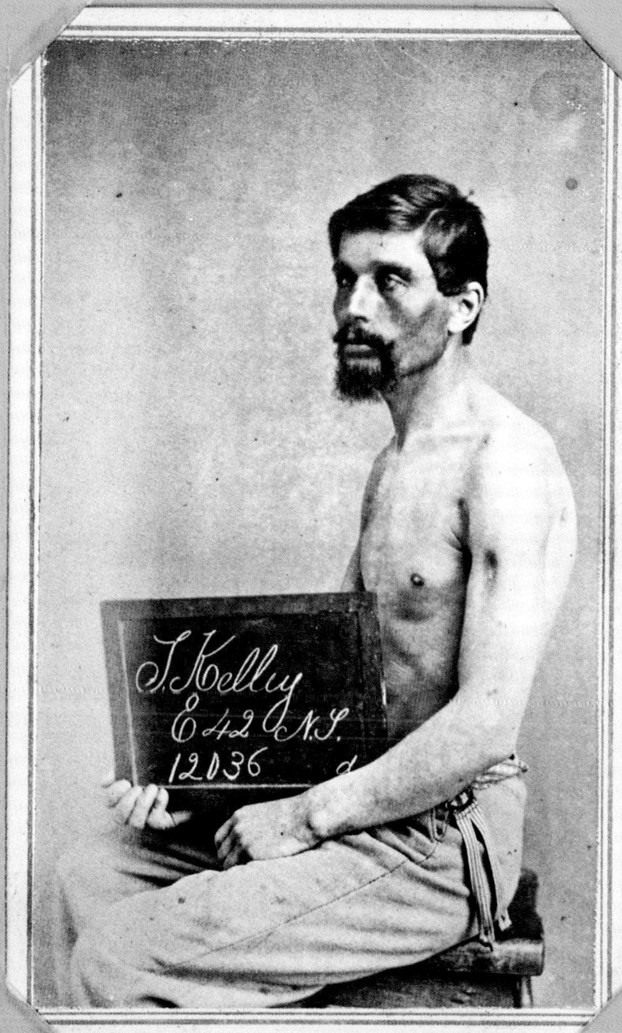

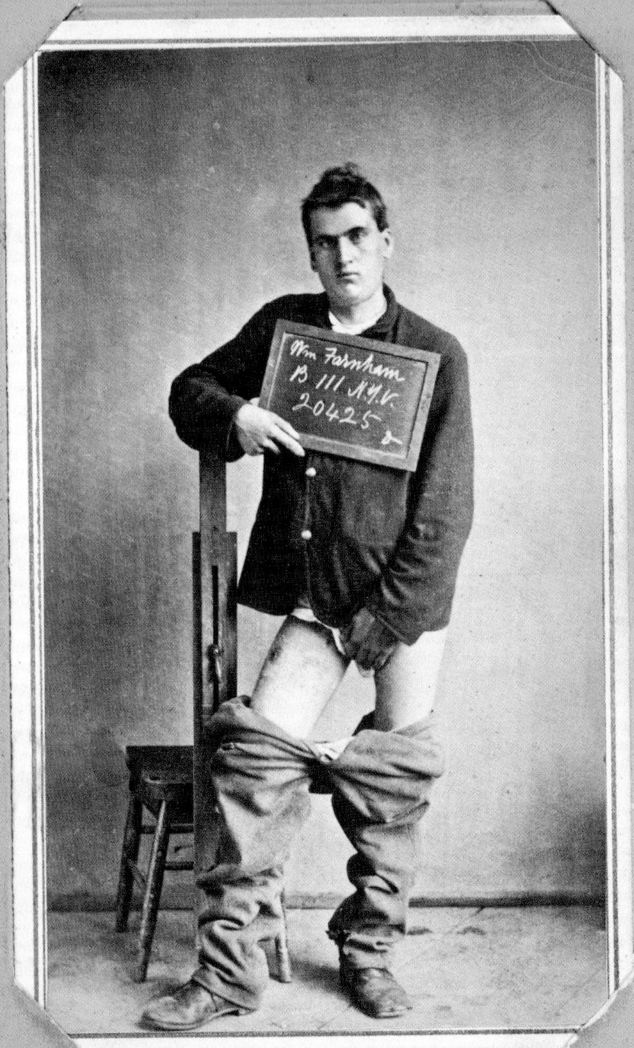

WILLIAM FARNHAM

CO B 111 NY

PETERSBURG

MARCH 30, 1865

GSW, RIGHT THIGH (FLESH).

DISCHARGED MAY 29, 1865

Aged 29, admitted to HH, Sept. 13th 1865. Wounded June 25, 1864. Operation performed at Lincoln Hospital. Soon after the parts became erysipelatous, extending through whole chest, gangrenous and sloughing, with destruction of soft parts the shaft was entirely removed by disarticulation at shoulder joint by straight incision on March 29th, 1865. The bone necrosed nine months after the amputation, several absesses collected in the stump. The patient is in good health, but with fistulous openings with considerable discharge of pus. Treatment disinfectant, astringent lotions.

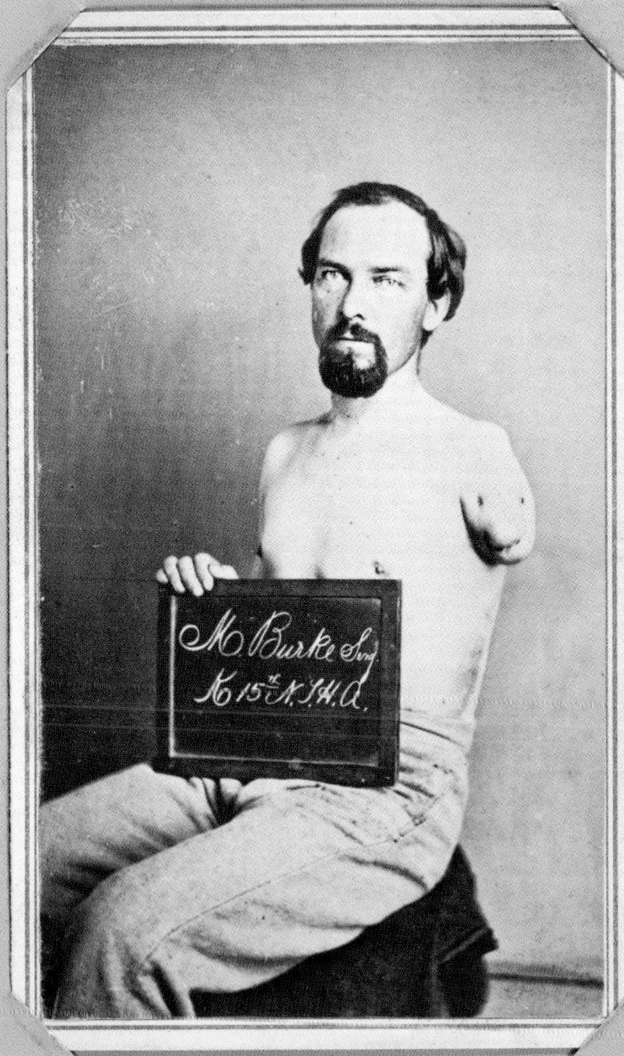

SGT. MARTIN BURKE

CO K 15 NY HA

PETERSBURG
JUNE 25, 1864

GSW, LEFT ARM.
AMPUTATION OF LEFT ARM AT SHOULDER.
WITH ERYSIPELAS (TREATED).

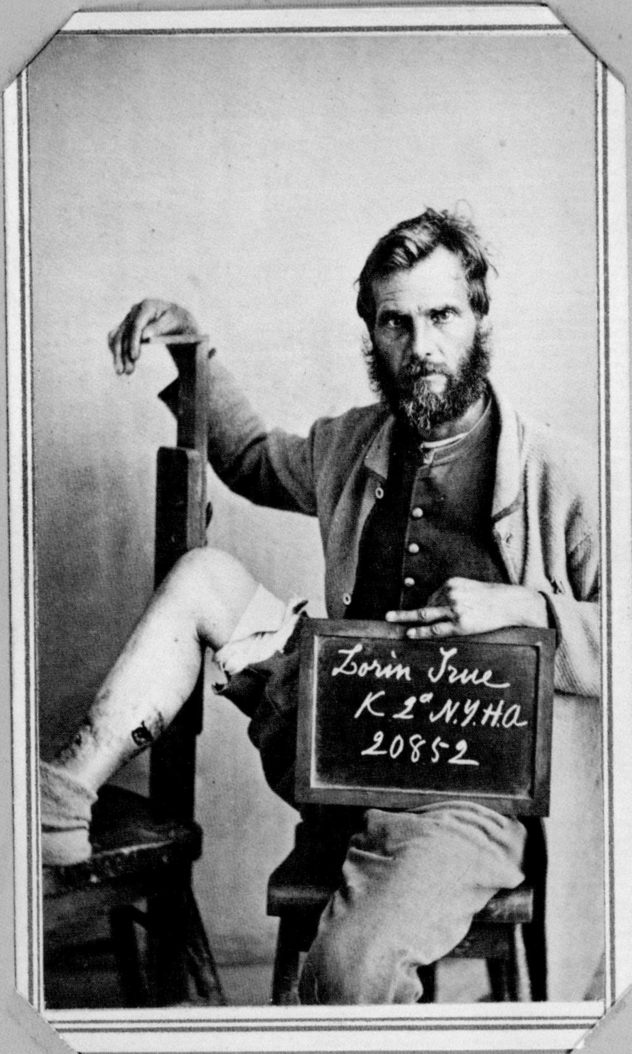

LORIN TRUE
CO K 2 NY HA

FARMERSVILLE
APRIL 7, 1865

GSW RIGHT LEG.

DISCHARGED JUNE 8, 1865

F. GUNDLACH
CO M 24 NY CAV

PETERSBURG
JUNE 17, 1864

GSW, RIGHT HAND.
AMPUTATION OF
THIRD FINGER.

DISCHARGED JULY 13, 1865

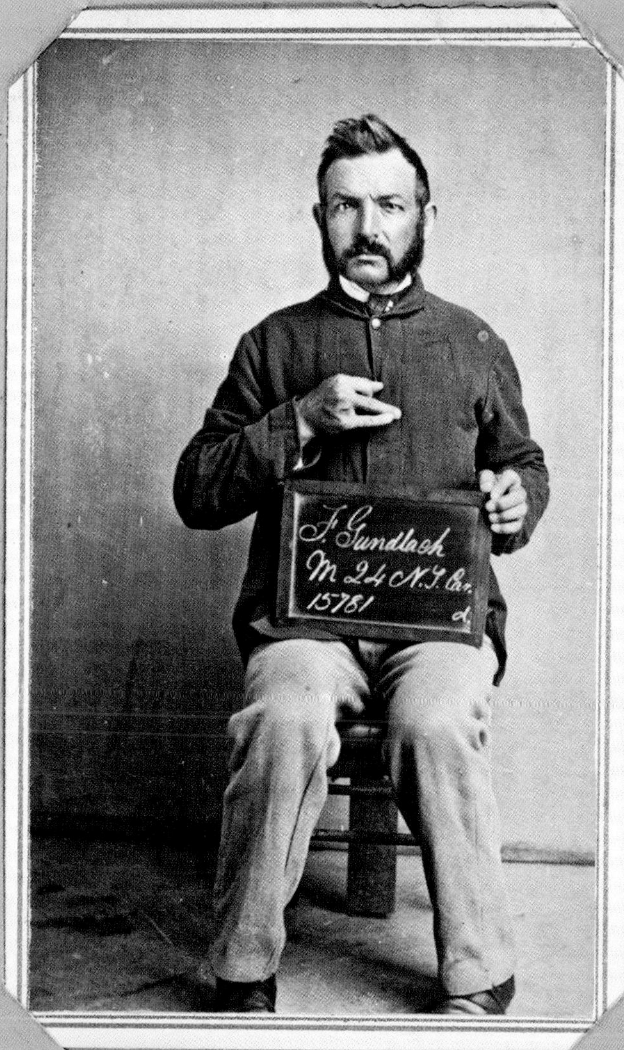

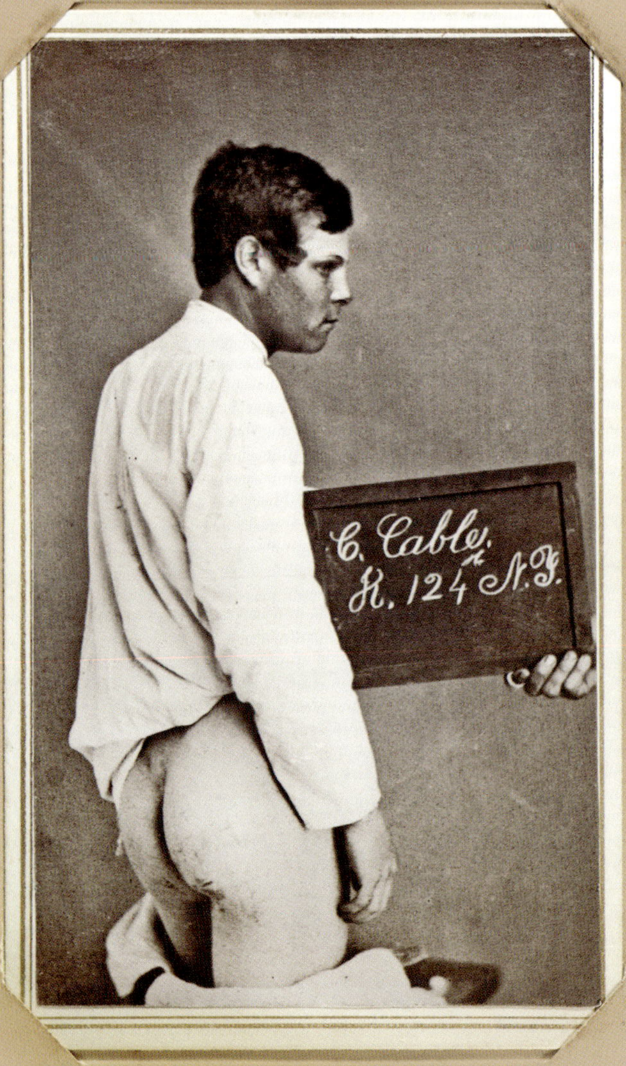

C. CABLE
CO K 124 NY

AMELIA COURT HOUSE
APRIL 6, 1865

GSW, LEFT THIGH.
UPPER THIRD EXIT GLUTIAL
MUSCLES, RIGHT SIDE.

DISCHARGED JUNE 8, 1865

CHARLES O'CONNER

CO K 155 NY

PETERSBURG

JUNE 22, 1864

GSW, LEFT ARM

DISCHARGED JUNE 22, 1865

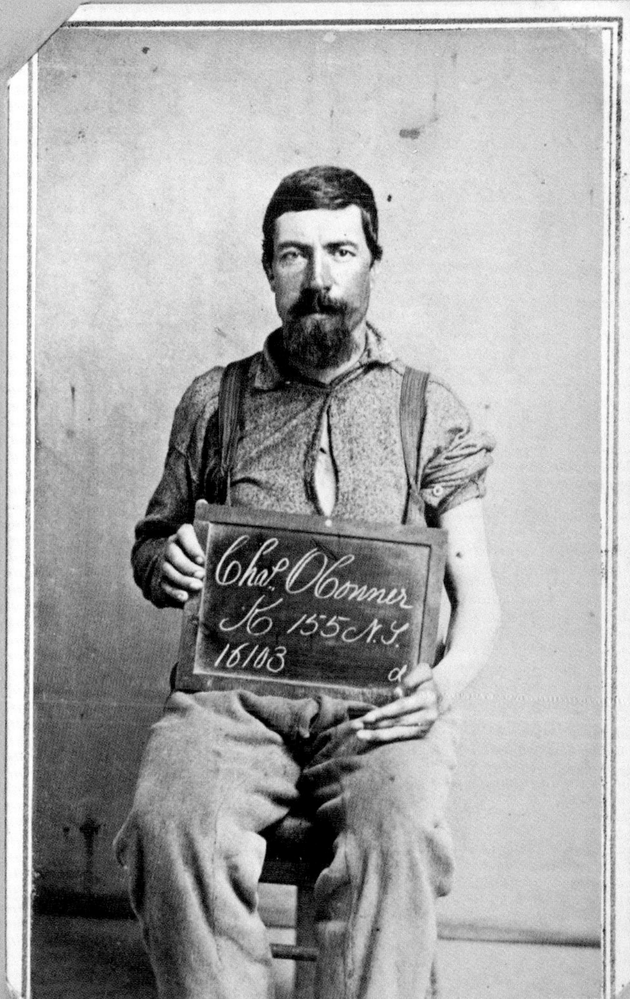

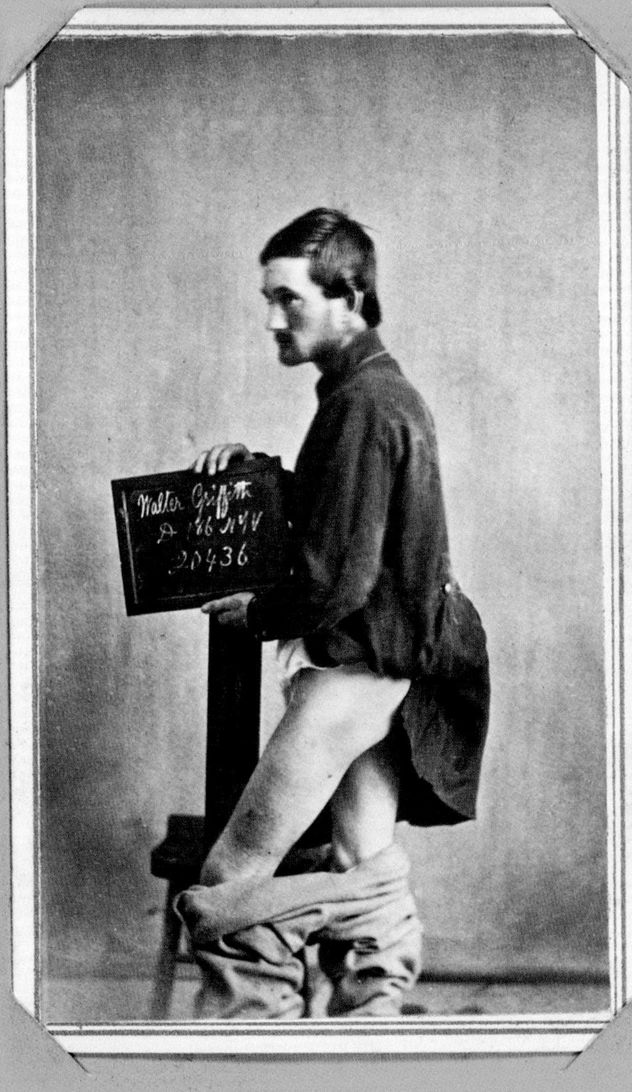

WALTER GRIFFITH
CO D 186 NY

PETERSBURG
APRIL 2, 1865

GSW, LEFT THIGH.

DISCHARGED MAY 29, 1865

31 years old. GSW left side near lumbar vertebra passing upward making its exit through the 9th and 8th ribs.

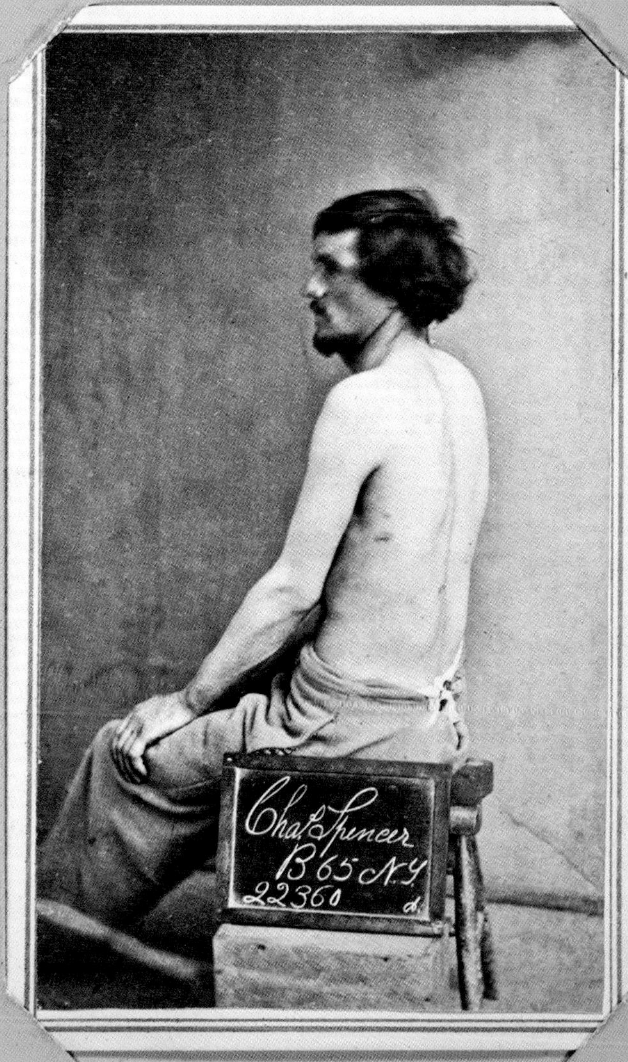

CHARLES SPENCER

CO B 65 NY

CITY CREEK

OCTOBER 19, 1864

GSW, LEFT SIDE.

TRANFRERRED JULY 20, 1865:
LINCOLN USA GEN HOSPITAL

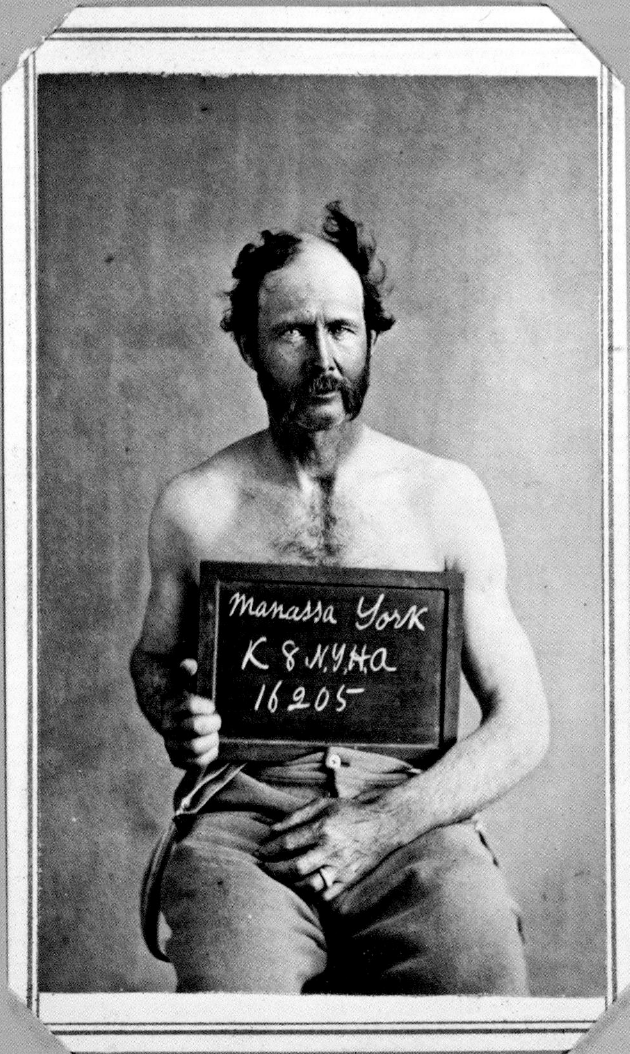

MANASSA YORK
CO K 8 NY HA

PETERSBURG
JUNE 17, 1864

GSW, LEFT ARM.

DISCHARGED MAY 29, 1865

G.R. OSMUN
CO E 69 NY

PETERSBURG
MARCH 28, 1865

GSW, LEFT LEG.

DISCHARGED JULY 5, 1865

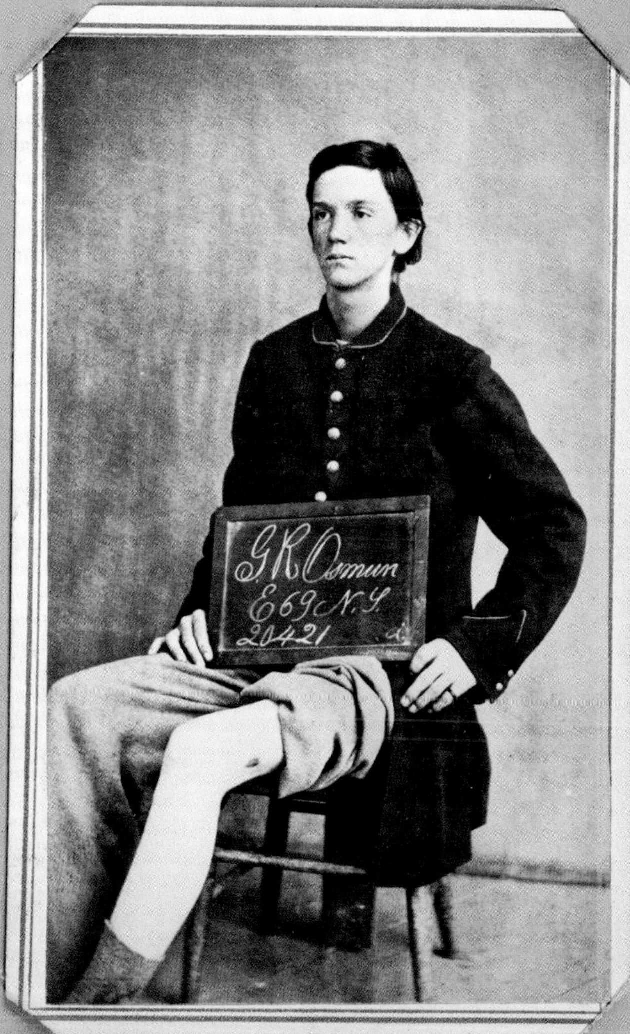

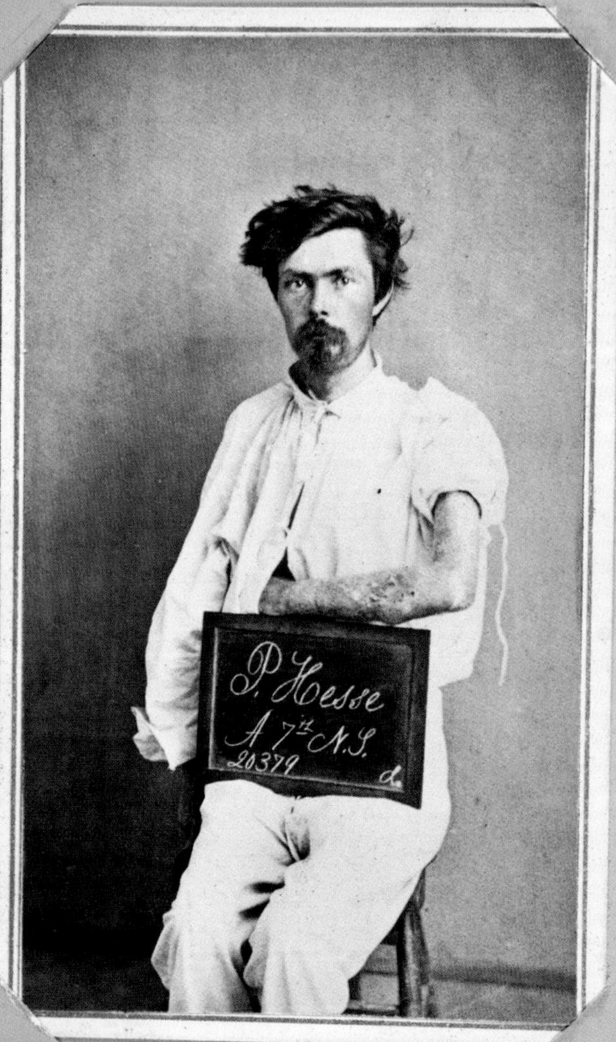

P. HESSE
CO A 7 NY

BOYDTON PLANK ROAD
(HATCHER'S RUN)
MARCH 31, 1865

GSW, LEFT ARM (FLESH).

RETURNED TO DUTY JULY 5, 1865

18 years old. GSW of forehead fracturing skull at Stone River TN, Dec 7, 1864. A farmer Considered totally disabled and Transferred to Hospital in Murfeesboro, TN. Dec 7, 1865. Bontecou declared him totally disabled for military service and one-third for civil occupation.

OHIO

JAMES COLETRAP

CO G 174 OH

STONE RIVER, TN
DECEMBER 7, 1864

GSW, HEAD.
DISABLED.

DISCHARGED JUNE 22, 1865

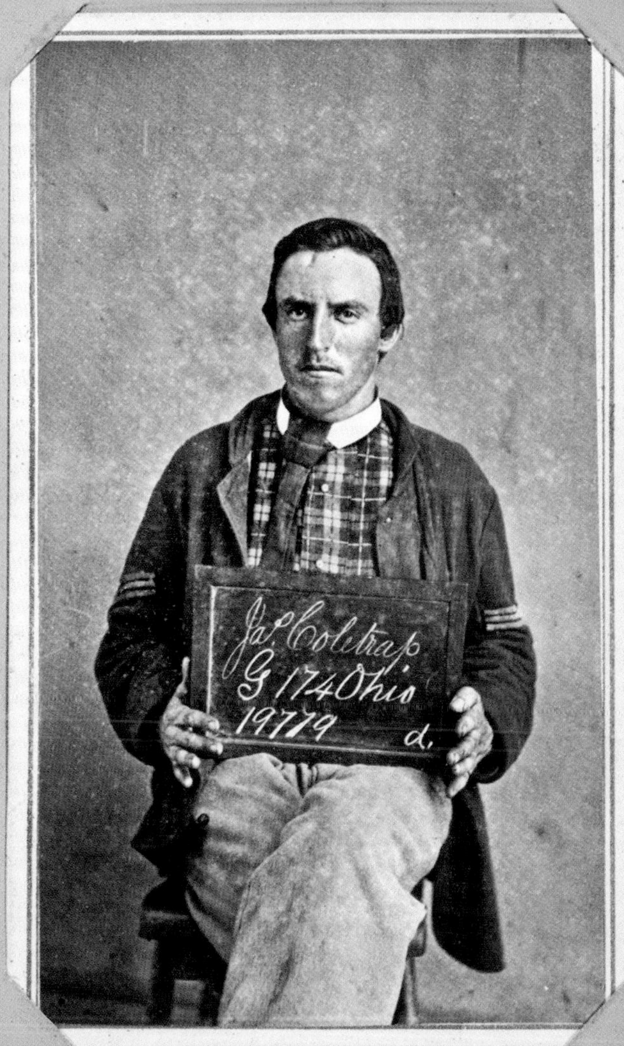

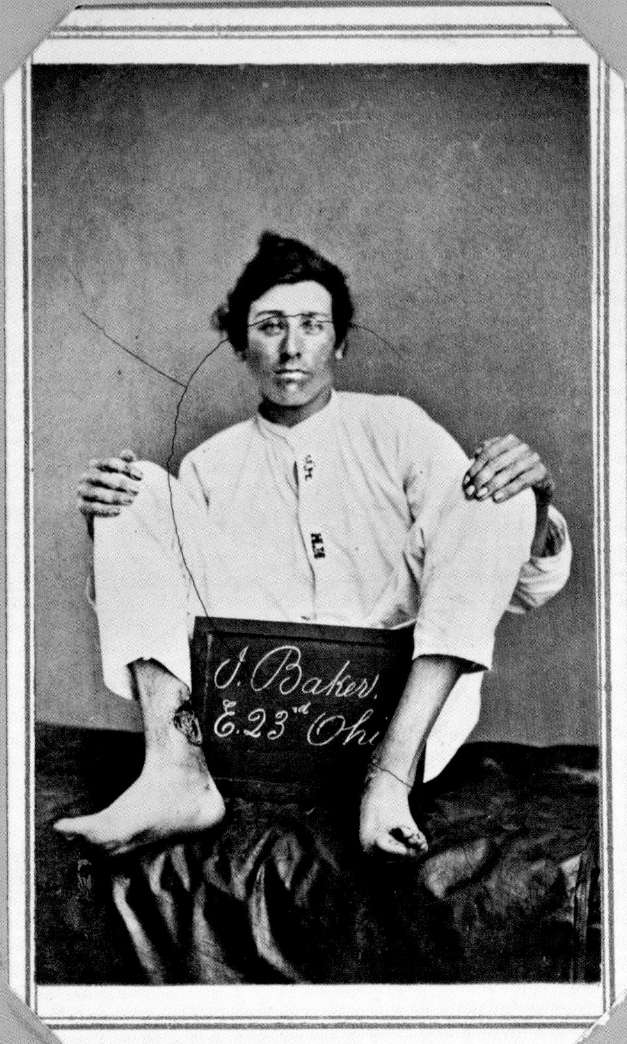

J. BAKER
CO E 23 OH

CHRONIC RHEUMATISM.
(GANGRENE)

TRANSFERRED MAY 18, 1865:
TO USA GEN HOSPITAL,
PHILADELPHIA

S. MIDDAGH
CO K 126 OH

WILDERNESS
MAY 6, 1864

GSW, LEFT SHOULDER.

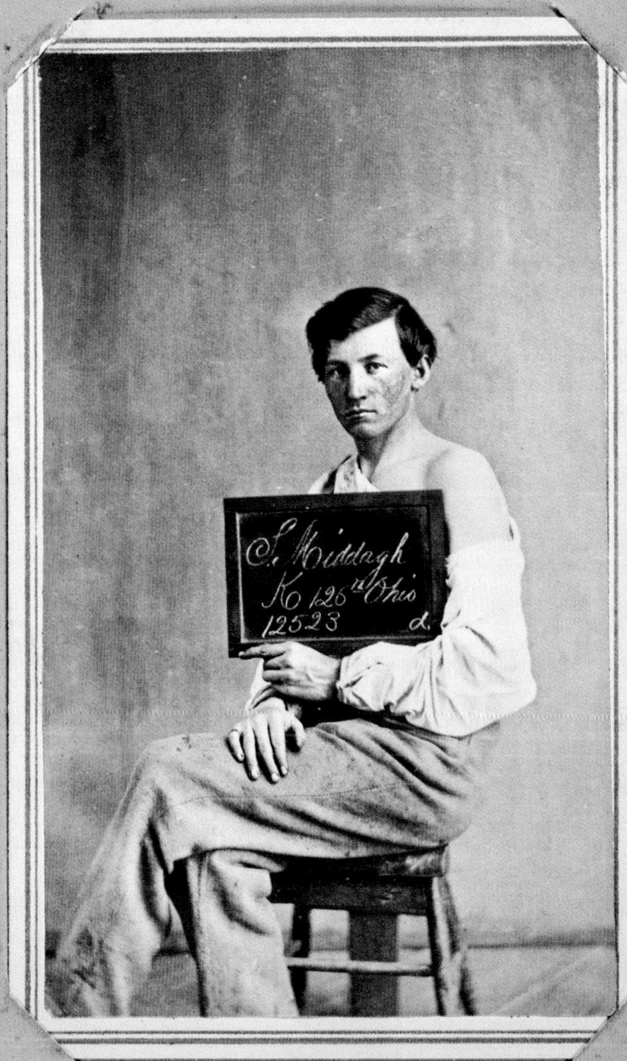

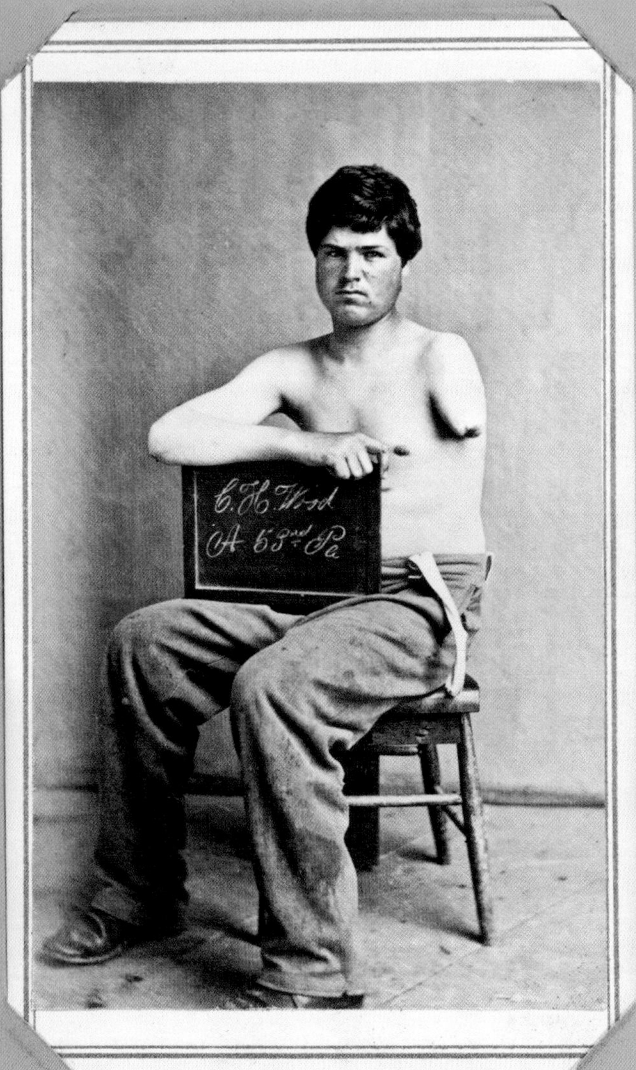

Aged 19, was admitted to HH, April 5, 1865, suffering from GSW of left arm, extent of injury unknown. Wounded March 31st at the Battle of Petersburg. The left arm was amputated on the field the same day by a circular incision. On admission, the stump was in good condition. Constitutional state of patient also good. Result favorable.

PENNSYLVANIA

C.H. WOOD

CO A 53 PA

PETERSBURG

MARCH 31, 1865

GSW, LEFT ARM.
CIRCULAR AMPUTATION
OF ARM, ON FIELD.

DISCHARGED JULY 6, 1865

Aged 43, admitted to HH, April 12, 1865, suffering from amputation of right thumb at metacarpal joint (bilateral flaps) result of GSW. Operation performed on field. The patient soon after admission, attacked with (phlegmonous) erysipelas. Large abscesses had formed in forearm, extending towards elbow joint, with great tumefaction of parts, but by deep and free incision and liberal internal use of ferric chloride and a nourishing supporting diet, the parts assumed a healthier appearance. Patient improving rapidly, parts entirely healed when patient was discharged.

J.B. SHADLE

CO C 87 PA

PETERSBURG

APRIL 2, 1865

GSW, RIGHT THUMB.
AMPUTATION
WITH ERYSIPELAS.

DISCHARGED JUNE 1, 1865

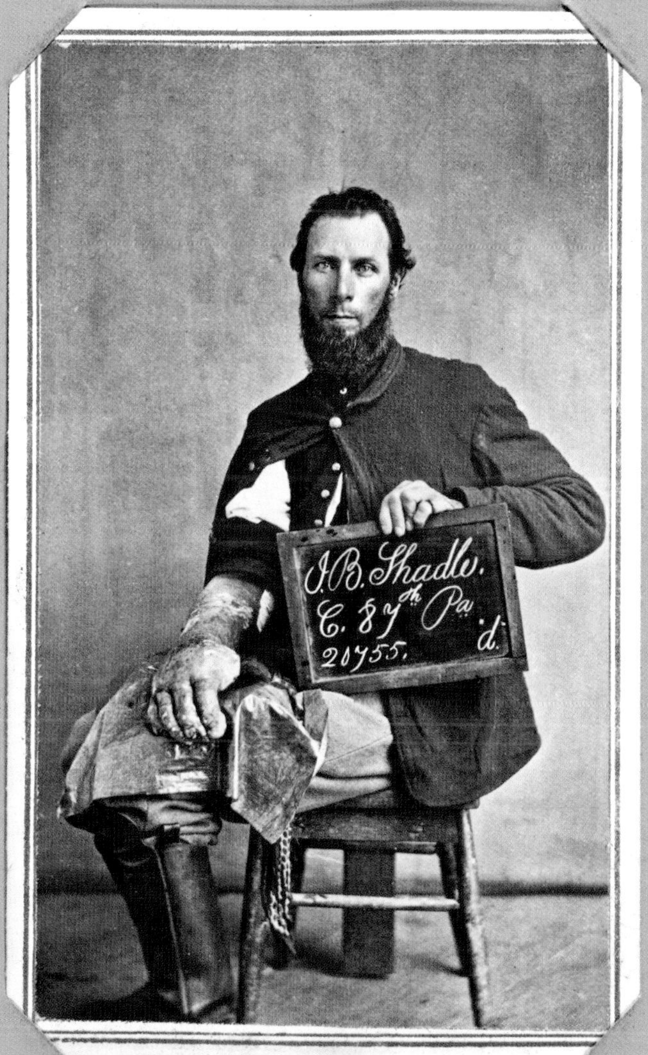

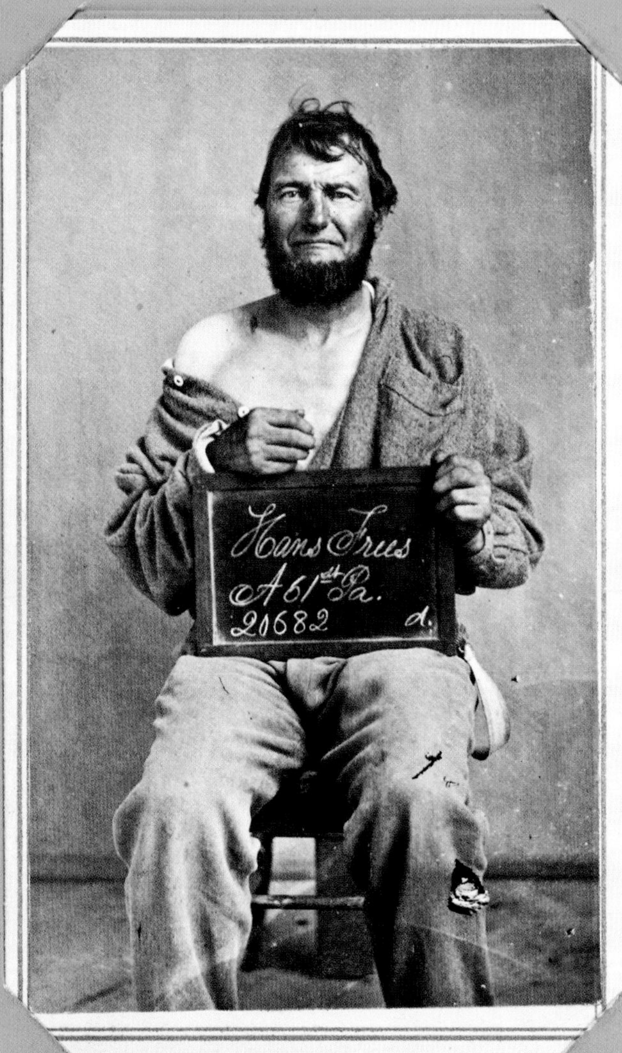

HANS FREES

CO A 61 PA

FORT FISHER

MARCH 28, 1865

GSW, RIGHT SHOULDER.

DISCHARGED JUNE 4, 1865

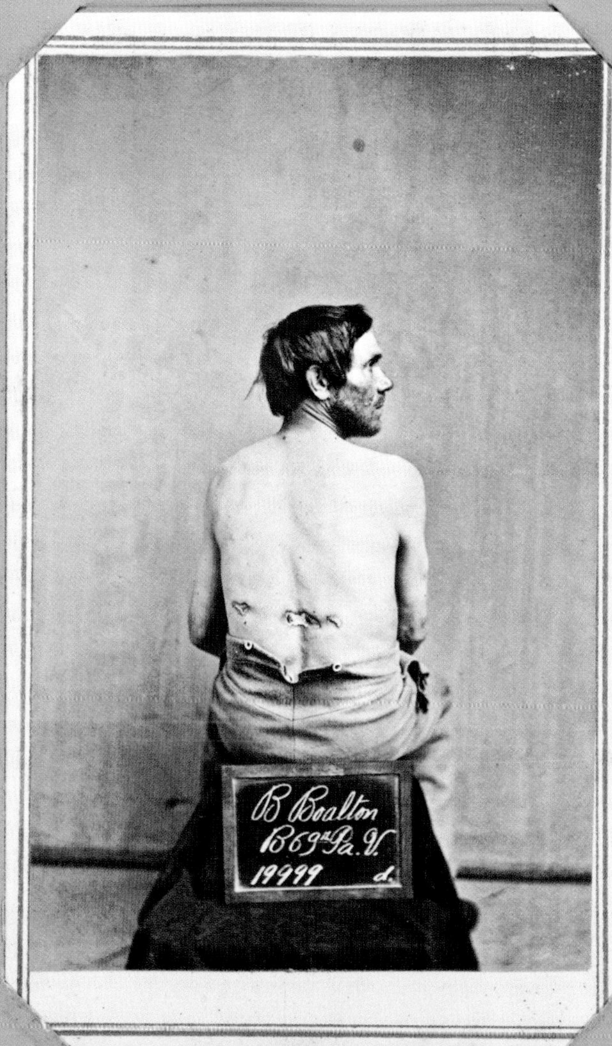

B. BOALTON

CO B 69 PA

HATCHER'S RUN

FEBRUARY 5, 1865

GSW, BACK DORSAL REGION.

DISCHARGED JULY 24, 1865

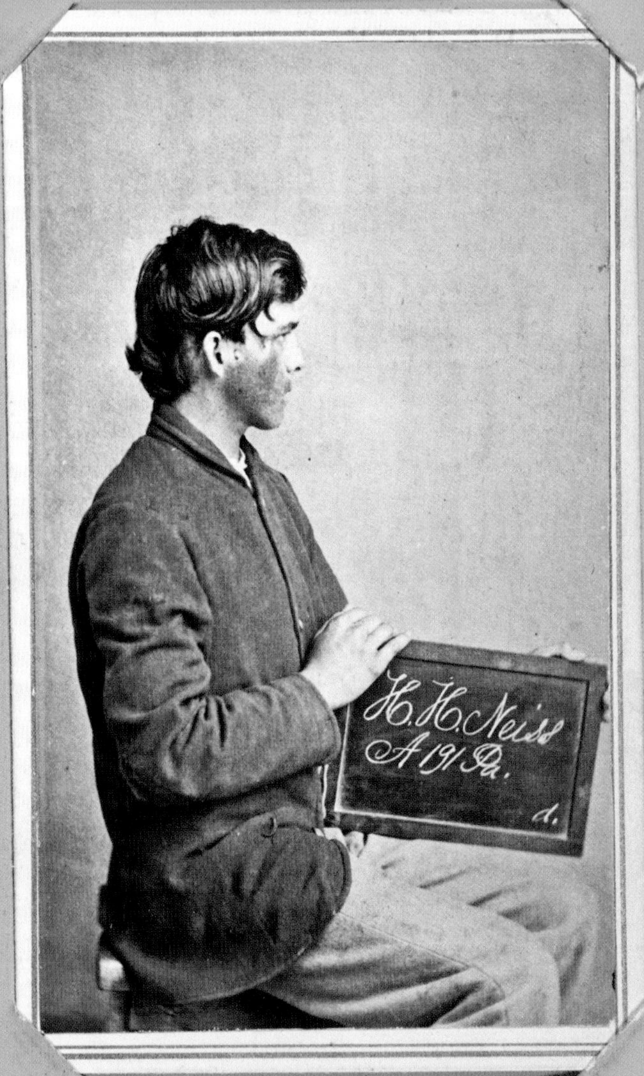

H.H. NEISS

CO A 191 PA

GSW, FACE.

DISCHARGED JULY 13, 1865

H. WILLIAMS

CO K 198 PA

APPOMATTOX COURT HOUSE, (THE DAY LEE SURRENDERED) APRIL 9, 1865

GSW, LEFT LEG & RIGHT FOOT. CIRCULAR AMPUTATION OF LEFT LEG & HAYS OPERATION ON RIGHT FOOT ON THE FIELD.

DISCHARGED OCT 6, 1865

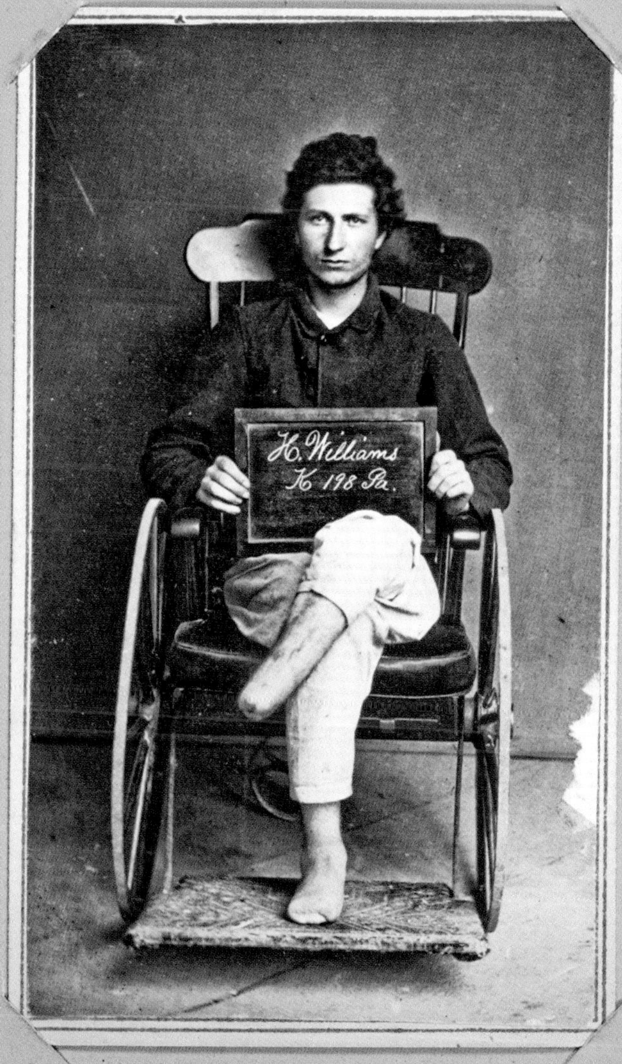

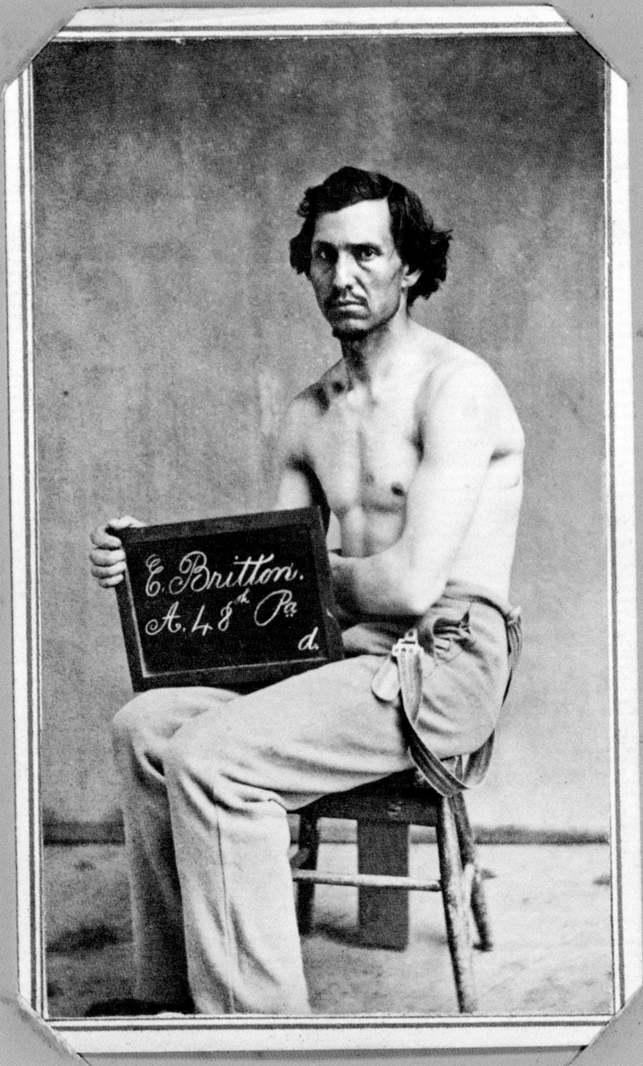

E. BRITTON
CO A 48 PA

PETERSBURG
JUNE 14, 1864

GSW, LEFT SIDE.

DISCHARGED JULY 24, 1865

A native of Poland, was admitted to HH November 2, 1865 with a circular amputation of the right thigh as a result of a GSW received at Petersburg March 31, 1865 while on picquet duty. Minie ball passed through the knee joint—was sent from field to City Point in 2 weeks, and thence to Douglas Hospital Wash. DC; where his thigh was amputated by Act'g Asst. Surgeon Haight, USA. Under ether, a sequestrum of bone four inches long was removed and several abscesses opened. Stump is now nearly healed.

MICHAEL SERABATSKY
CO B 183 PA

PETERSBURG
MARCH 31, 1865

GSW, THROUGH RIGHT KNEE.
AMPUTATION OF THIGH.

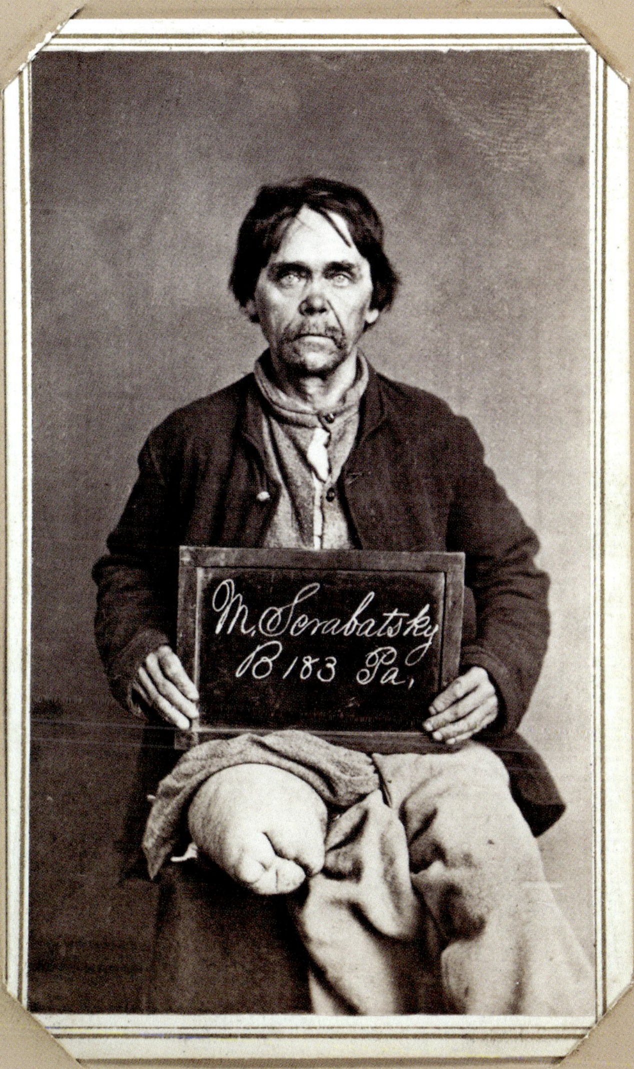

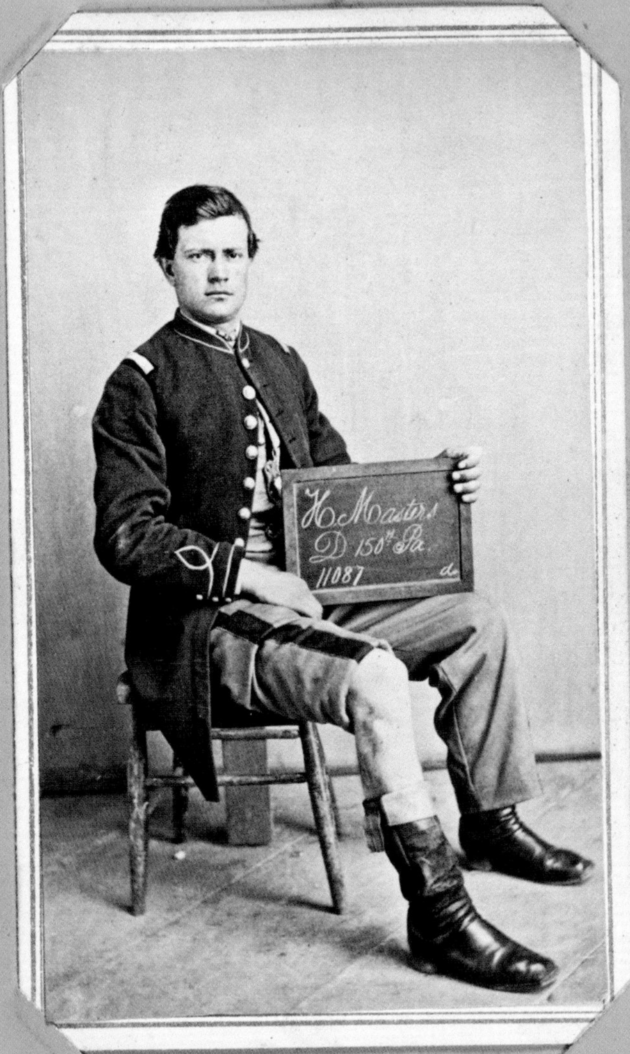

H. MASTERS

CO D 150 PA MUSICIAN

GSW, RIGHT LEG.

DISCHARGED MAY 27, 1865

20 years old. Enlisted as laborer, GSW and fracture of the forearm received at Charlestown VA: Bontecou declared him totally disabled for military service and one-third for civil occupation.

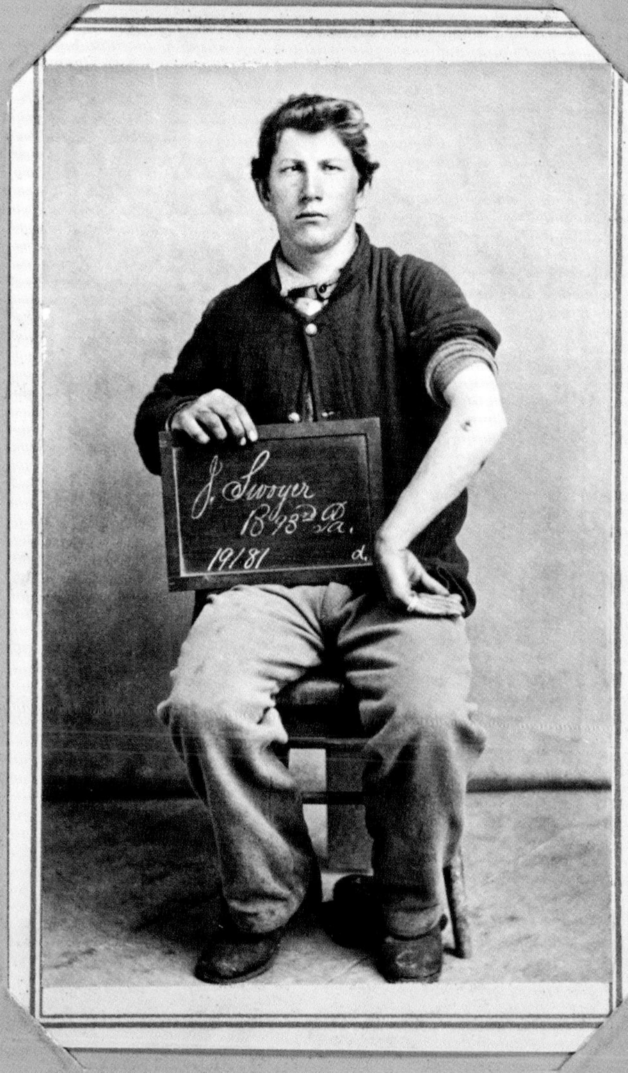

JACOB SWOYER

CO B 93 PA

CHARLESTON

AUGUST 21, 1864

GSW, FRONT LEFT ARM, UPPER THIRD, FRACTURING ULNA.

DISCHARGED JUNE 1, 1865

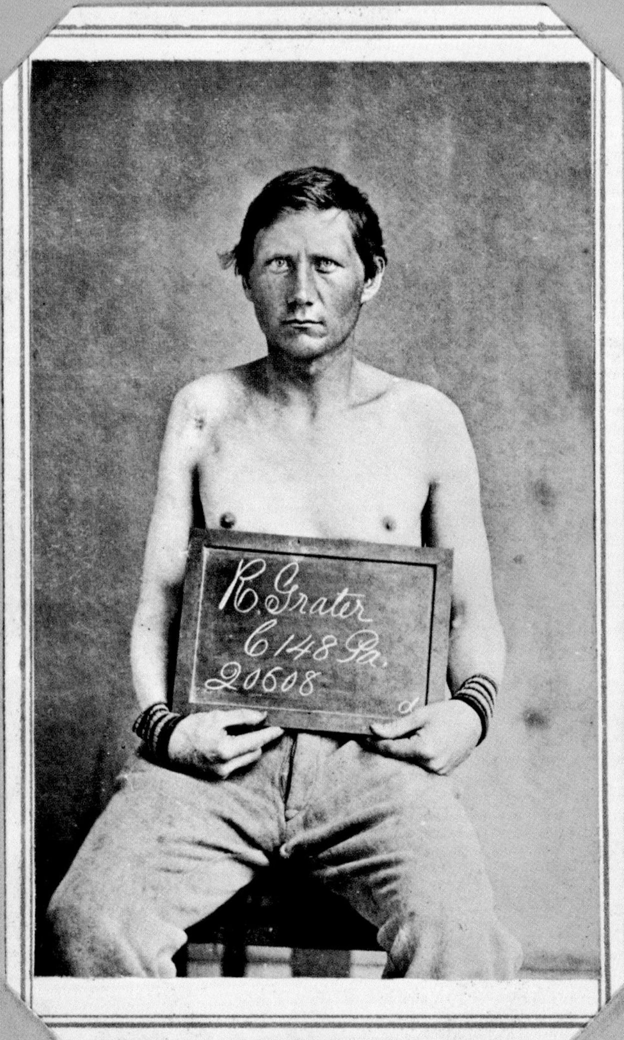

R. GRATER

CO C 148 PA

CHANCELLORSVILLE

MAY 3, 1864

GSW, RIGHT SHOULDER.

DISCHARGED JULY 23, 1865

S. FRANKENBERGER
CO D 1 PA CAV

PETERSBURG
OCTOBER 9, 1864

GSW, FRONT RIGHT HAND.

DISCHARGED JUNE 22, 1865

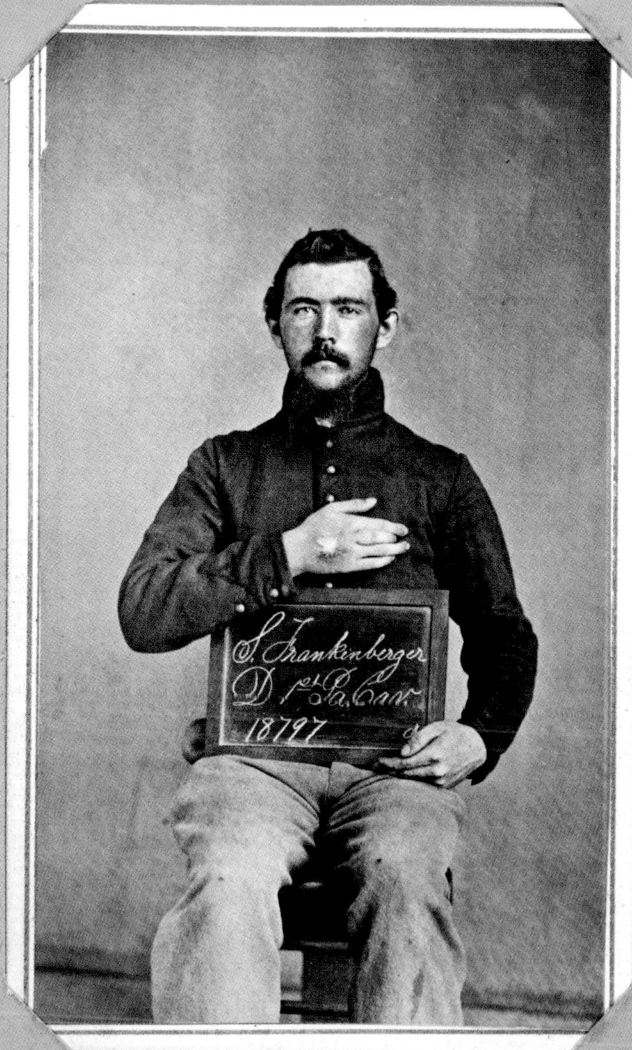

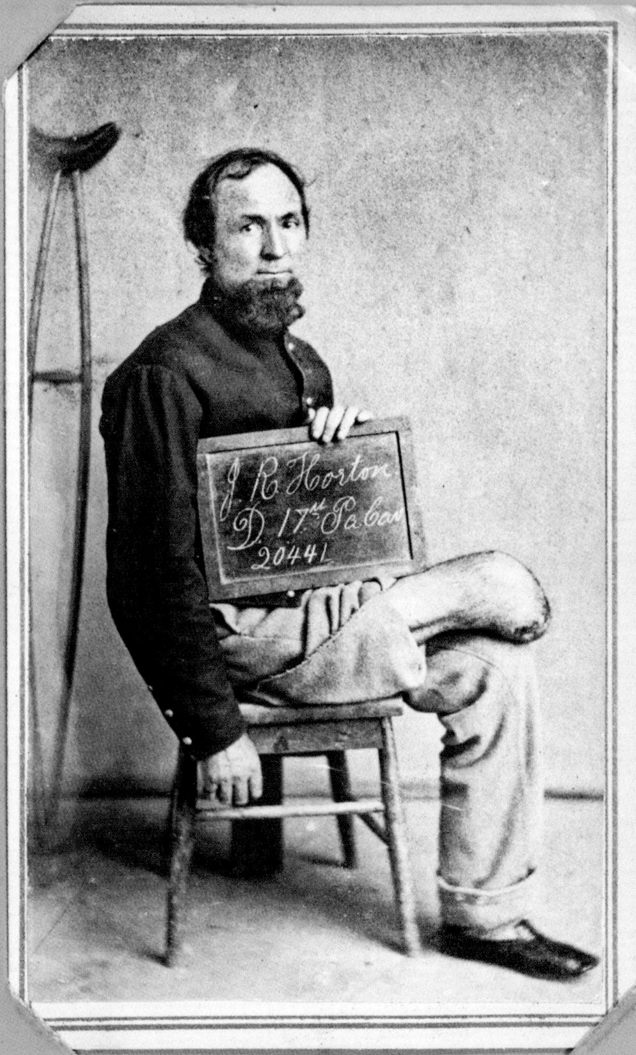

Aged 41 years, admitted to HH April 5, 1865, suffering from GSW of right leg. Wounded March 31 at Battle of Petersburg. Amputation of right leg upper thigh, anteroposterior flaps, on field, April 2, 1865. On admission constitutional state of patient was good. Result favorable. Doing well.

JOSEPH R. HORTON

CO D 17 PA CAV

PETERSBURG

MARCH 31, 1865

GSW, RIGHT LEG.
AMPUTATION AT UPPER THIRD
WITH ANTEROPOSTERIOR
FLAPS, ON THE FIELD.

TRANSFERRED JULY 20, 1865:
LINCOLN USA GEN HOSPITAL

J.W. HOLLEN
CO J 205 PA

PETERSBURG
APRIL 2, 1865

GSW, RIGHT WRIST.

DISCHARGED JUNE 21, 1865

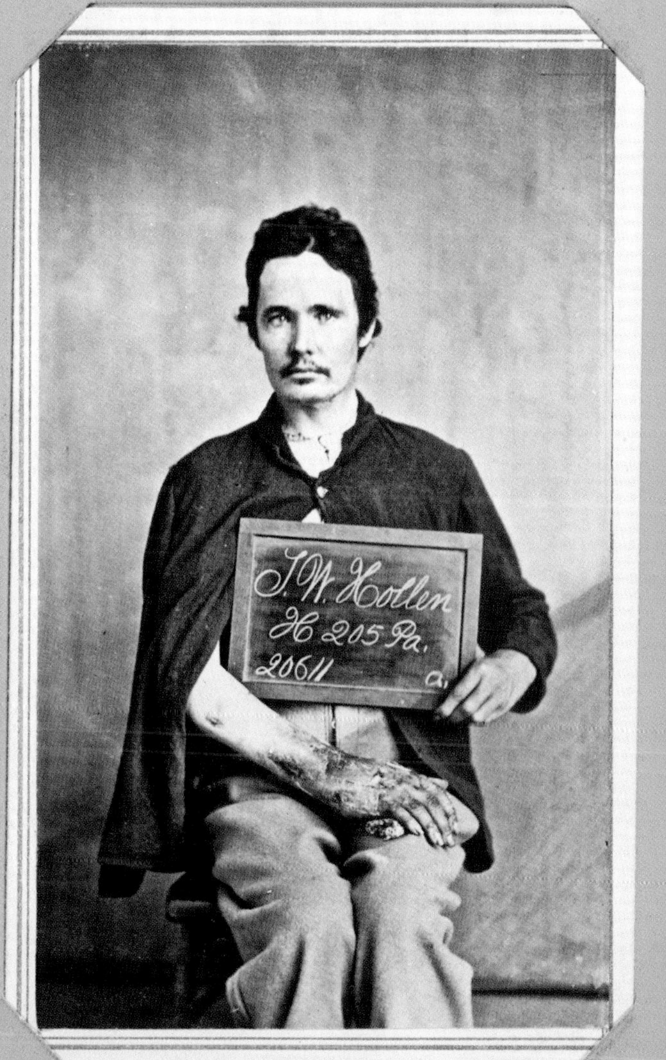

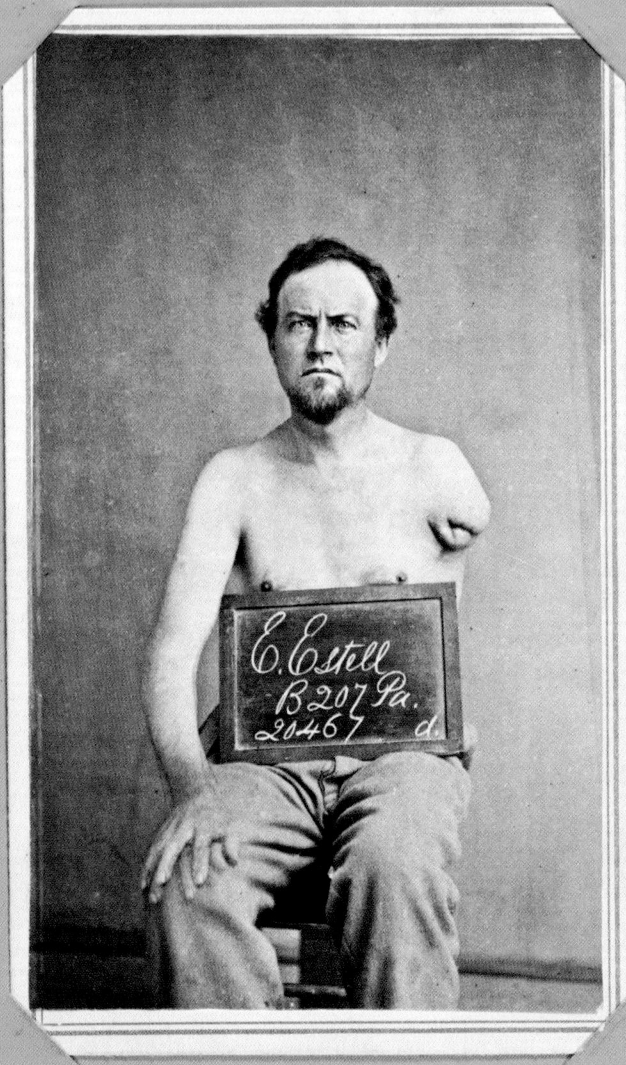

Disability report of 1884 notes he "never wore an artificial limb" as the amputation was too near the joint and the area still remains very tender.

EDWARD ESTELL

CO B 207 PA

PETERSBURG

APRIL 2, 1865

GSW, LEFT ARM
AMPUTATION LEFT ARM, UPPER THIRD ANTERIOR/ POSTIEROR FLAPS.

DISCHARGED JULY 13, 1865

J.G.VALE
CO K 200 PA

PETERSBURG
MARCH 25, 1865

GSW, LEFT GROIN.

DISCHARGED JULY 10, 1865

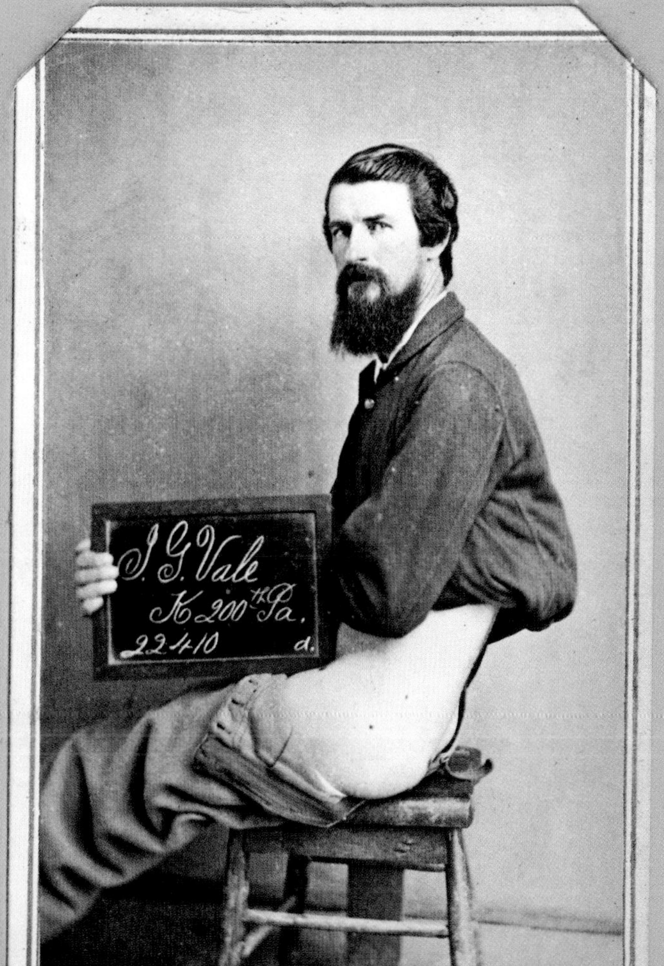

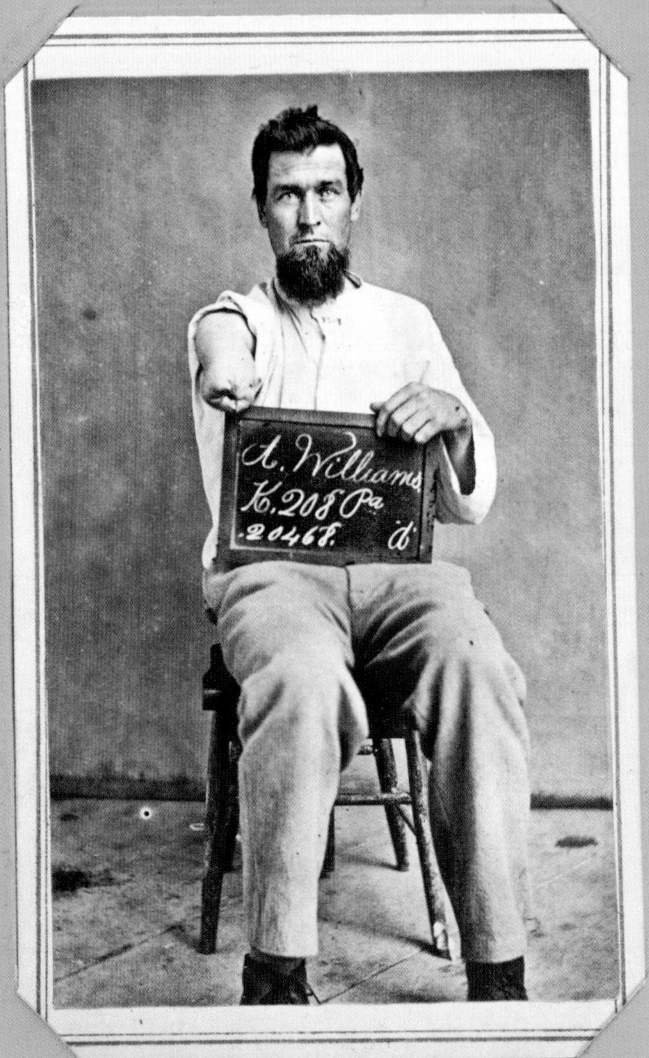

Williams, aged 38, was discharged from HH on Bontecou's certificate of disaility. Notes: 'loss of right arm by amputation... in consequence of which he is totally disabled for military service and for civil occupation wholly.'

ALVAH R. WILLIAMS

CO K 208 PA

PETERSBURG
MEADE STATION
APRIL 2, 1865

GSW, RIGHT ARM.
CIRCULAR AMPUTATION OF RIGHT ARM MIDDLE THIRD, ON THE FIELD.

DISCHARGED JUNE 8, 1865

Aged 41, admitted to HH, March 23rd, 1865 with accidental gunshot wound of the left hand. The ball entered about the middle of the palmar surface, and emerged at the dorsal, fracturing the third metacarpal bone. The wound was received near Petersburg, Va., March 15th 1865, and was caused by the conoidal ball. The use of the middle finger is much impaired, in consequence of the necessary removal of loose spicula of bone, and gangrenous sloughing of tendon of flexor muscle. The patient had erysipelas in the left arm a short time, but yielded promptly to treatment. The wound has entirely healed.

JOSEPH BRIGGS

CO D, 8 PA CAV

PETERSBURG
MARCH 15, 1865

GSW, LEFT HAND.

DISCHARGED JUNE 23, 1865

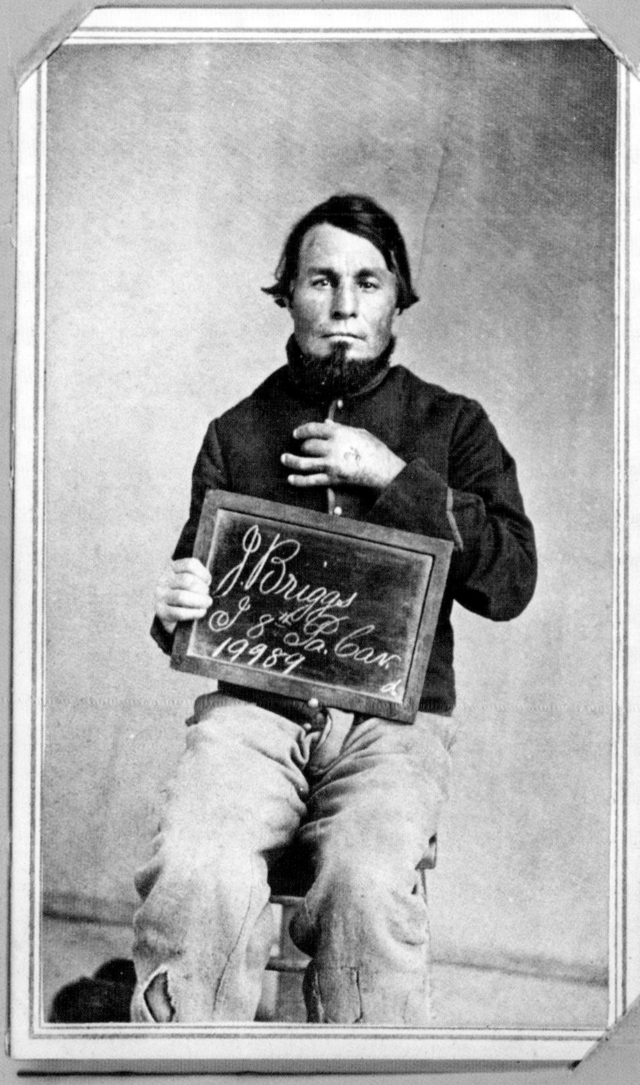

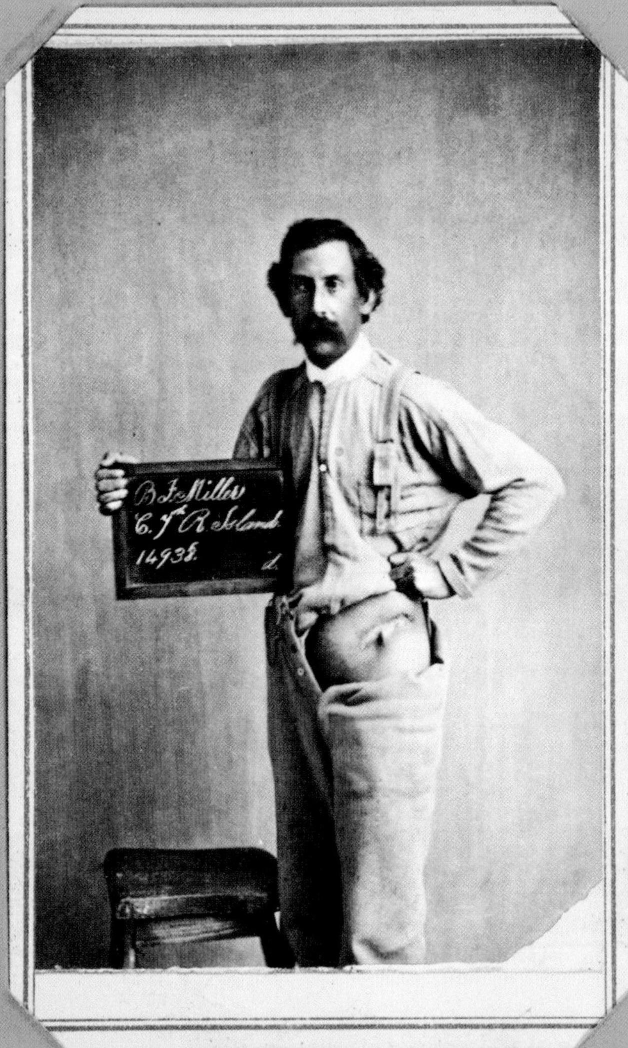

RHODE ISLAND

B. F. MILLER
CO C 7 RD

COLD HARBOR
JUNE 3, 1864

GSW, LEFT HIP.

DISCHARGED MAY 25, 1865

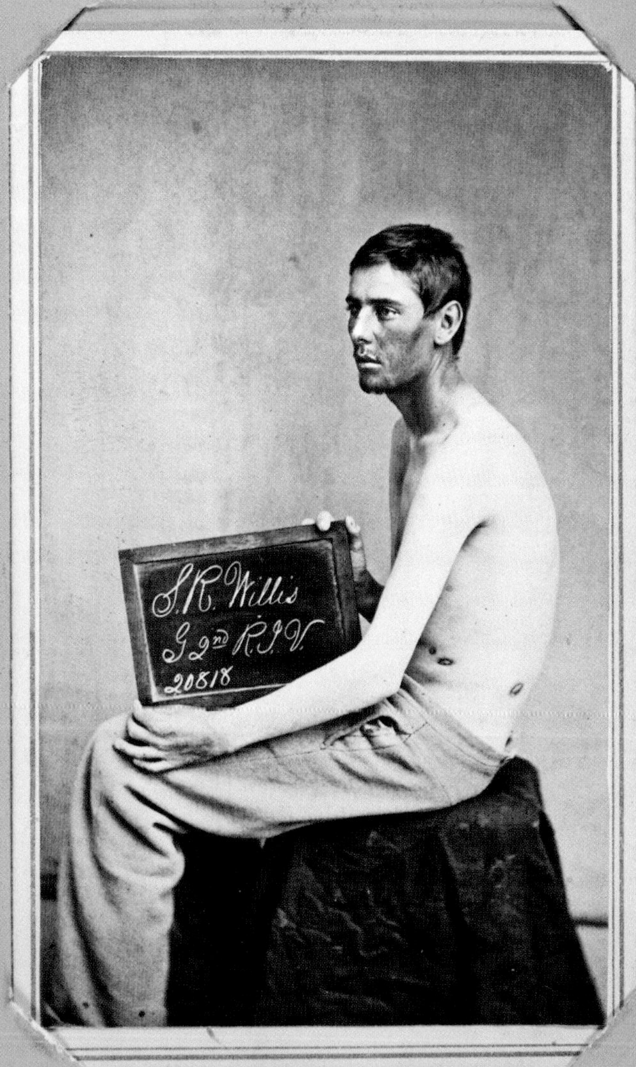

S. R. WILLIS
CO G 2 RI

FARMERSVILLE
APRIL 6, 1865

GSW, LEFT SIDE.

DISCHARGED JULY 24, 1865

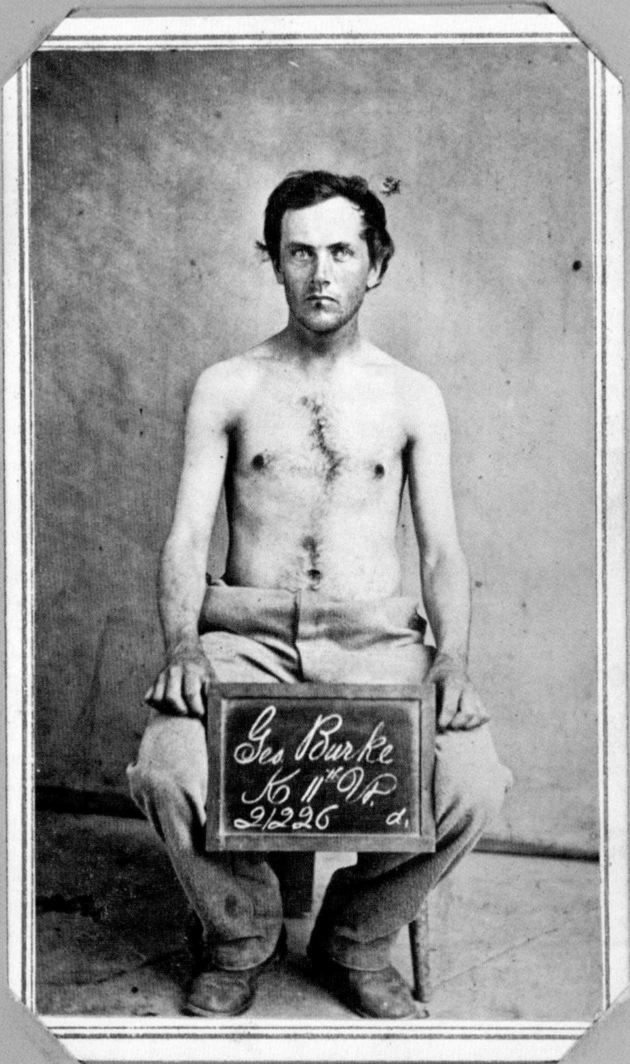

VERMONT

GEORGE BURKE

CO K 11 VT

GSW, CHEST.

J. S. BOSWELL
CO E 1 VT CAV

PETERSBURG
APRIL 1, 1865

GSW, LEFT THIGH.

TRANSFRERED APRIL 20,1865:
USA GEN HOSPITAL,
MONTPILLIER

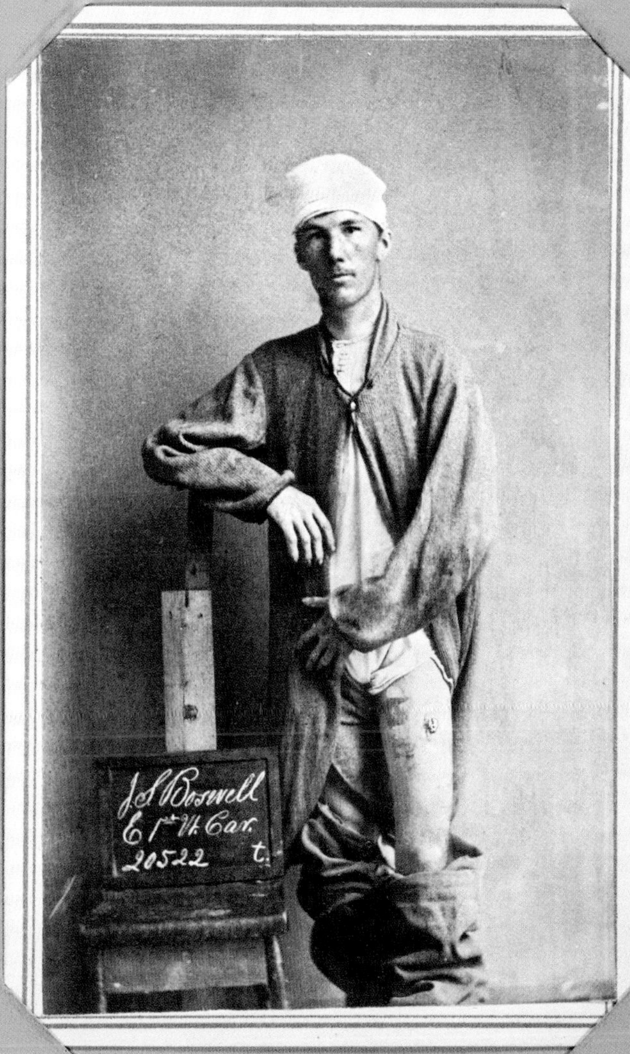

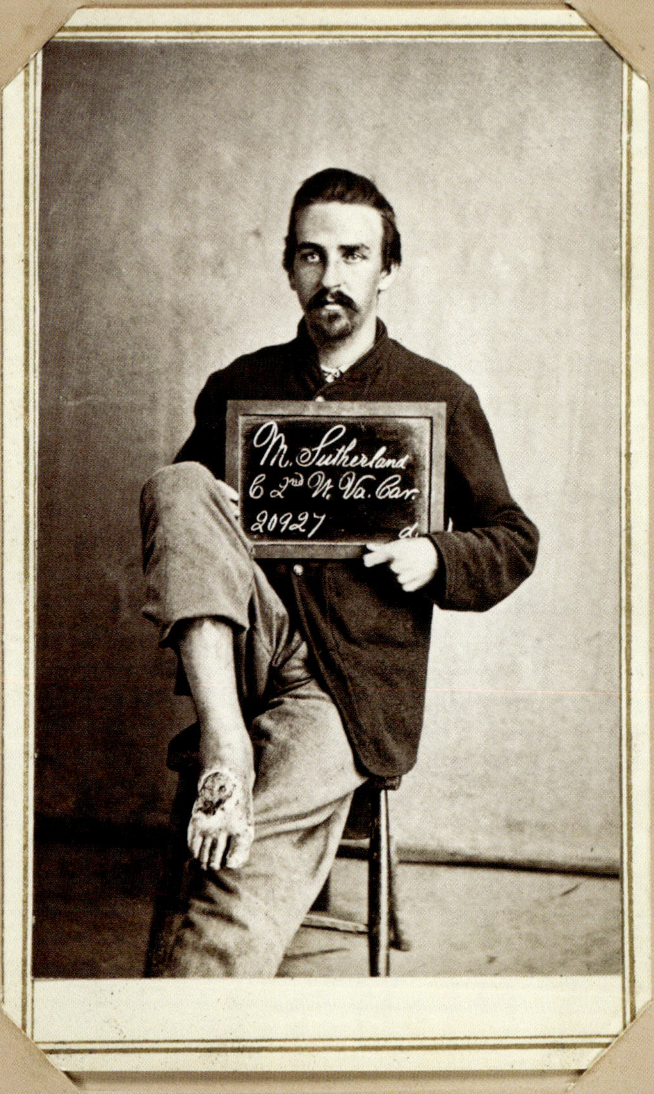

WEST VIRGINIA

M. SUTHERLAND
CO C 2 W VA CAV

APPOMATTOX
APRIL 8, 1865

GSW, RIGHT FOOT.

DISCHARGED JULY 24, 1865

30 years old. GSW right clavicle and neck Wounded May 12, 1864 Spotsylvania. Bontecou declared him totally disabled for military service and one-third for civil occupation. Declared disabled one-third for manual occupation.

Decker was captured at the Second Battle of Bull Run, Aug. 29, 1862 and released on a prisoner trade Sept. 3, 1862.

WISCONSIN

MOSES DECKER

CO D 6 WIS

SPOTSYLVANIA

MAY 12, 1864

GSW, RIGHT SHOULDER.

DISCHARGED JULY 28, 1865

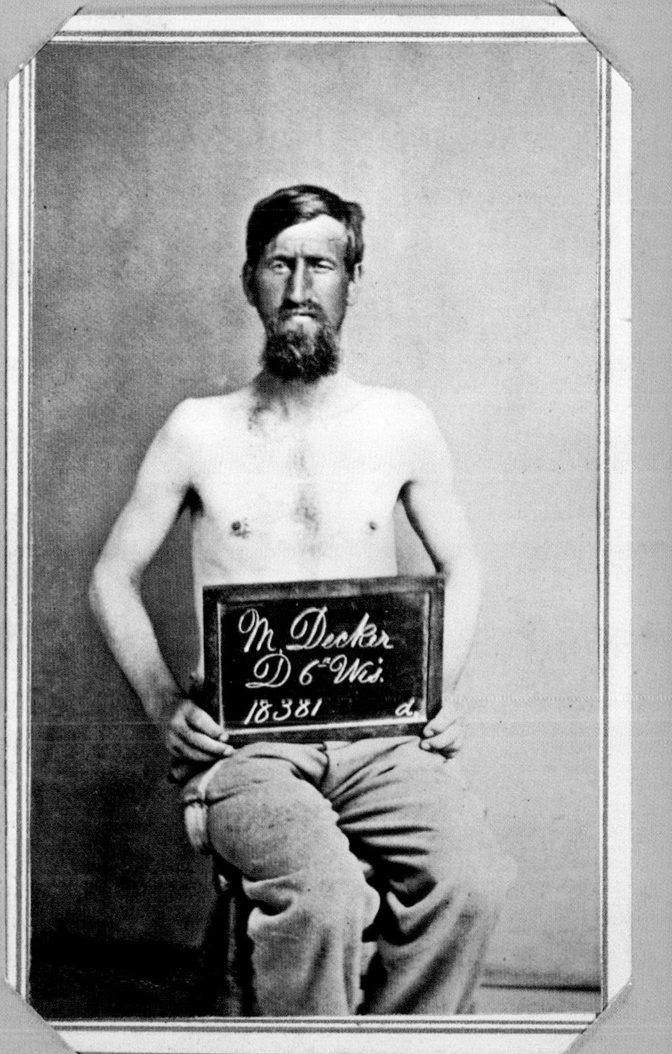

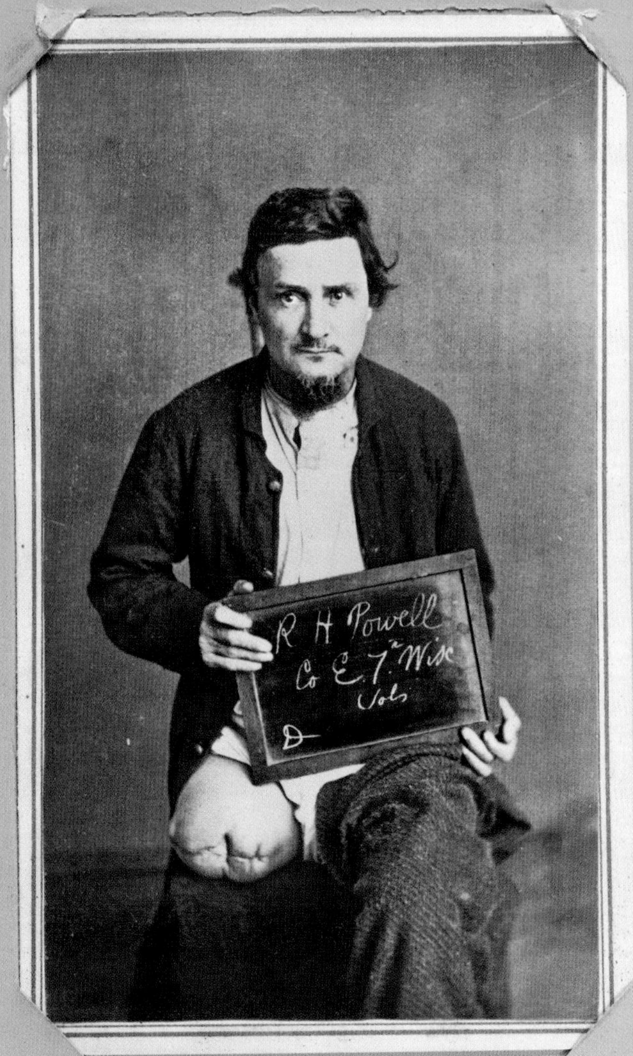

ROBERT H. POWELL
CO E 7 WIS

SOUTH SIDE RAIL ROAD
MARCH 31, 1865

GSW RIGHT THIGH.
AMPUTATION AT THIGH.

DISCHARGED NOV 28, 1865

N. HAMMOND
CO K 5 WIS

HIGHHILL
APRIL 6, 1865

GSW, LEFT LEG.

TRANSFERRED JULY 20, 1865:
LINCOLN USA GEN HOSPITAL

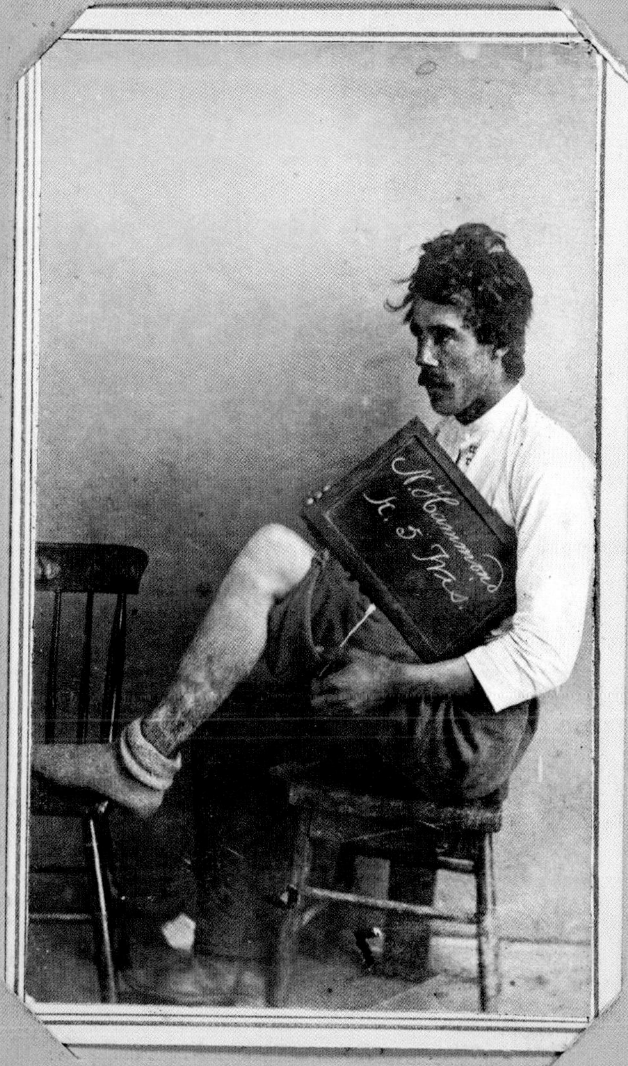

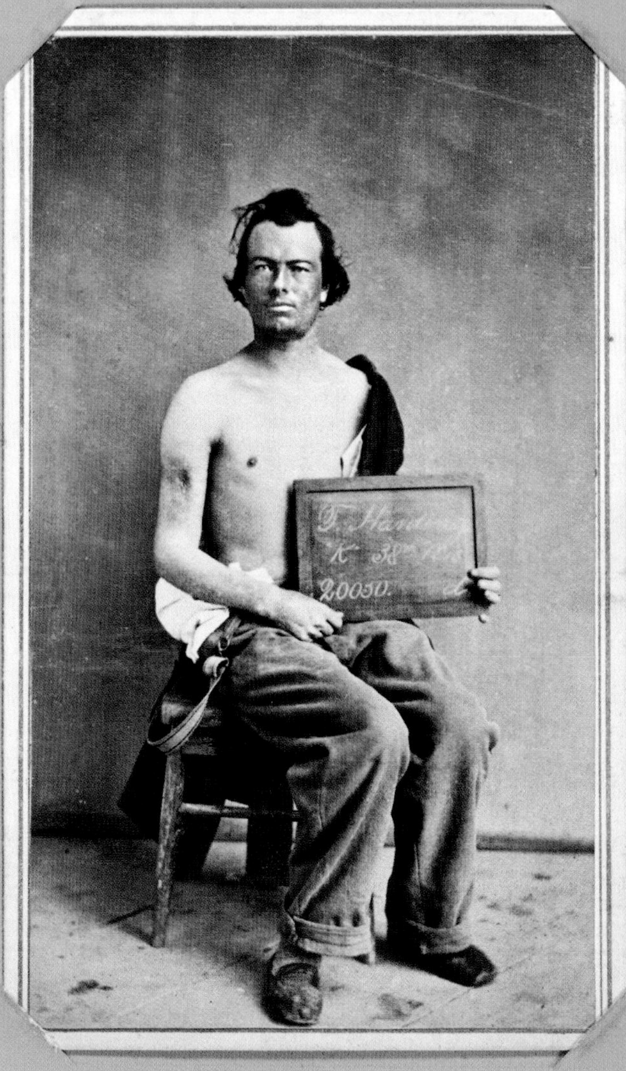

F. HARDING

CO K 38 WIS

HATCHER'S RUN

MARCH 4, 1865

SHELL WOUND, HUMERUS.
RESECTION OF UPPER THIRD.
ONE INCH OF BONE REMOVED,
OPERATION ON THE FIELD.

DISCHARGED JUNE 19, 1865

Age 19, admitted to HH, April 19, 1865, with GSW of the chest. The ball entered about midway between the right nipple and the sternum, passed transversely and emerged about a half inch external to the left nipple. It was supposed there was slight injury of some of the thoracic contents. Percussion and auscultation normal in the right chest. Slight dullness on percussion [sic] of the left side; respiration nearly normal. The patient preferred the recumbent posture, as sitting up or moving about, caused pain. He was apparently well, except for pain on motion. The pericardium was supposed to be penetrated by the ball.

F. GROSS

CO F 5 WIS

SAYLER'S CREEK

APRIL 6, 1865

GSW, CHEST.

DISCHARGED JULY 4, 1865

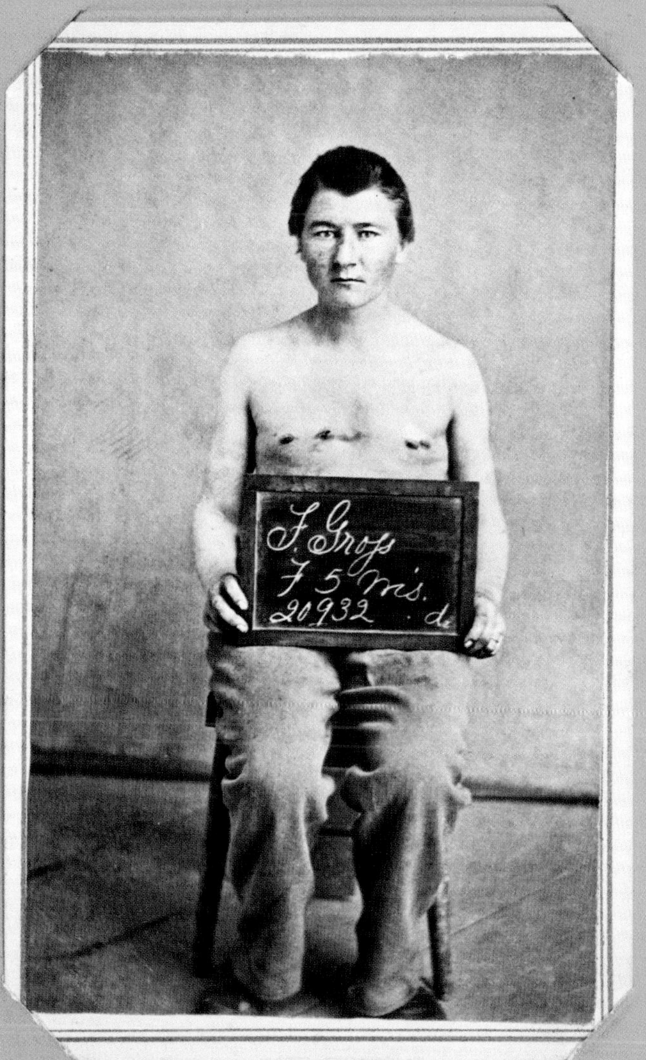

THE BATTLES

WILDERNESS MAY – JUN 1864

NAME	UNIT	PLATE
Boyce, S.	Co B 5 MI	24
Kelly, J.	Co E 42 NY	60
Lanning, H.	Co C 86 NY	40
Middagh, S.	Co K 126 OH	74

SPOTSYLVANIA MAY 1864

NAME	UNIT	PLATE
Brower, H.	Co C 10 NY Zou	36
How, G.	Co B 122 NY	54
Decker, M.	Co D 6 WI	98

COLD HARBOR MAY 1864

NAME	UNIT	PLATE
Emery, S.	Co B 5 NH	28
Gilkey, H.	Co H 13 NH	29
Johnson, W.	Co D 2 NH	31
Miller, B.	Co C 7 RI	93

PETERSBURG- SIEGE MAY – NOV 1864

NAME	UNIT	PLATE
Britton, F.	Co A 48 PA	81
Burke, M.	Co K 15 NY HA	62
Dillon, R.	2 Bat Vrc	5
Frankenberger, S.	Co D 1 PA Cav	86
Felder, L.	CO F 11 MA Bat	21
Garrison, G.	Co A 95 NY	50
Gunlach, F.	Co M 24 NY Cav	64
Harris, C.	Co A 31 US Col	4
Howland, N.	Co E 58 MA	22
Johnson, C.	Co G 120 NY	55
O'Conner, C.	Co K 155 NY	66
York, M.	Co K 8 NY HA	69

PETERSBURG- APPOMATTOX MAR – APR 1865

NAME	UNIT	PLATE
Armsrtong, J.	Co K 1 SC	1
Artel, H.	Co B 2 MD	18
Boswell, J.	Co E 1 VT Cav	96
Botswick, E.	Co H 2 NY Cav	45
Briggs, J.	Co D 8 PA Cav	92
Church, F.	Co D 1 NY Cav	58
Cross, G	Co M 4 NY HA	39
Delahan, B.	Co J 8 LA	2
Estell, E.	Co B 207 PA	89
Farnham, W.	Co B 111 NY	61
Fonger, P.	Co K 1 MI Cav	23
Foss, F.	Co 4 ME Bat	16
Gillespie, C.	Co F 94 NY	43
Greenfield, C.	Co F 79 NY HA	FP
Griffith, W.	Co D 186 NY	67
Hollen, J.	Co J 205 PA	88
Horton, J.	Co D 17 PA Cav	87
Jollife, J.	Co K 116 PA	FC
Martin, H.	Co H 8 NJ	35
Murphy, P.	Co B 11 ME	13
Osmun, G.	Co E 69 NY	70
Serabatsky, M.	Co B 183 PA	82
Sargent, C.	Co C 1 ME HA	15
Shadle, J.	Co C 87 PA	76
Talbot, A.	Co A 14 NY HA	59
Templeton, D.	Co A 46 NY	37, 38
Van Valkenburgh, E.	Co C 39 IL	10
Vale, J.	Co K 200 PA	90
Wilson, H.	Co F 106 NY	41
Williams, A.	Co K 208 PA	91
Wood, C.	Co A 53 PA	75

KEY: INFANTRY: INF. CAVALRY: CAV, HEAVY ARTILLERY: HA, UNITED STATES COLORED TROOPS: US COL. VETERAN'S RESERVE CORPS: VRC, VOLUNTEER: VOL, ZOUAVE: ZOU, BATTERY: BAT, MUSICIAN: MUS.

HATCHERS RUN FEB – APRIL 1865

NAME	UNIT	PLATE
Boalton, B.	Co B 69 PA	78
Fryer, R.	Co G 52 NY	52
Harding, F.	Co K 38 WI	101
Mather, C.	Co K 1 MI Cav	27
Russell, R.	1 DE	9
Van Schaack, J.	Co K 125 NY	53

SOUTH SIDE RAILROAD MARCH – JUNE 1865

NAME	UNIT	PLATE
Lone, P.	Co H 64 NY	47
Powell, R.	Co E 7 WI	99
Secord, J.	Co H 5 MI Cav	26
Smith, A.	Co G 69 NY	42

FARMERSVILLE APRIL 1865

NAME	UNIT	PLATE
Beam, A.	Co J 26 MI	25
True, L.	Co K 2 NY HA	63
Willis, S.	Co G 2 RI	94

APPOMATTOX APRIL 1865

NAME	UNIT	PLATE
Sutherland, M.	Co C 2 WV Cav	97
Williams, H.	Co K 198 PA	80
Weller, R.	E 7 MD	17

MISC BATTLES

NAME	UNIT	PLATE
Cable, C.	Co K 124 NY	65
Coletrap, J.	Co G 174 OH	72
Coombs, L.	Co K 4 US Inf	3
Cunard, C.	Co A 7 NJ	33
Frees, H.	Co A 61 PA	77
Gates, A.	Co G 188	46
Grater, R.	Co C 148 PA	85
Gross, F.	Co F 5 WI	102
Hammond, N.	Co K 5 WI	100
Hesse, P	Co A 7 NY	71
Hunter, G.	Co A 1 NJ Cav	34
Kitchell, E.	Co K 15 NJ	32
Knight, J.	Co D 111 IL	12
Miller, J.	Co K 56 NY	57
Murphy, J.	Co K 37 MA	19
Swoyer	Co B 93 PA	84
Spencer, C.	CO B 65 NY	68
Stokes, J.	Co H 185 NY	49
True, L.	Co K 2 NY HA	63

NO BATTLE LISTED

NAME	UNIT	PLATE
Burke, G.	Co K 11 VT	95
Folsom, J.	Co D 6 NH	30
Masters, H.	Co D 150 PA Mus	83
Neiss, H.	Co A 191 PA	79
Rich, D.	Co C 10 VRC	6
Seal, M.	Co D 28 IL	11

DISEASE (NOT IN BATTLE)

NAME	UNIT	PLATE
Ashen, M.	Co H 9 NY Cav	48
Baker, J.	Co E 23 OH	73
Dorsey, M.	Co D 14 CT	8
Hemenway, O.	10 VRC	7
Parker, A.	Co D 1 ME Cav	14
Reynolds, B.	Co C 154 NY	56
Robinson, D.	Co B 151 NY	44
Swift, H.	Co 21 MA	20
Watson, J.	Co G 164 NY	51

PRIMARY REFRENCES

Adams, George Worthington. *Doctors in Blue: The Medical History of the Union Army in the Civil War*. New York: Henry Schuman, 1952.

Burns, Stanley. *Civil War Medical Photography*. New York: Burns Archive, 1980/3.

Cunningham, H.H. *Doctors in Grey: The Confederate Medical Service*. Baton Rouge: Louisiana State University Press, 1958.

Faust, Drew Gilpin. *This Republic of Suffering: Death the American Civil War*. New York: Alfred A. Knopf, 2008.

Freemon, Frank. *Microbes and Minie Balls: An Annotated Bibliography of Civil War Medicine.* London and Toronto: Associated University Presses, 1993.

Henry, R.S. *The Armed Forces Institute of Pathology: Its First Century, 1862-1962*. Washington, DC: Government Printing Office, 1964.

Kelley, H. and W. Burrage. *Dictionary of American Medical Biography*. New York: Appleton & Co., 1928. (p. 1208).

Macdonald, John. *The Historical Atlas of the Civil War*. New York: Chartwell Books, Inc., 2010.

Weeks, Michael. *The Complete Civil War Road Trip Guide.* Woodstock, VT: The Countryman Press, 2009.

Whitman, Walt. *Specimen Days & Collect*. Philadelphia: David McKay, 1882-83.

ONLINE RESOURCES:

Heritage Preservation Services with the National Park Service
http://www.nps.gov/history/hps/abpp/civil.html

New York State Military History Museum
www.dmna.state.ny.us/historic/reghist/CWN.html

The State of New York and The Civil War
www.nycivilwar.us/

U.S. Army Heritage & Education Center
www.ahco.army.mil/

ACKNOWLEDGMENTS

First and foremost I would like to thank Lissa Rivera whose artistic talents helped create this book as well as the Archive 'Gem Series.' National Museum of Health & Medicine personnel Dr. Marc Micozzi, Michael Rhode and Kathleen Stocker provided 25 years of research assistance. Collectors and dealers who helped me over the years include Joseph Buberger, Clifford & Michele Krainik, Wes Cowan and William Gladstone. Museum curators provided guidance in appreciating Bontecou's art, especially Jeff Rosenheim, Metropolitan Museum of Art, Tom Beck, Albin O. Kuhn Gallery, UMBC, as well as Michael McAfee and Michael Winey of US Army Archives. The dedicated staff at The Burns Archive—Sarah Simms and Alice Dana provide constant support and research that facilitate my publications.

OTHER BOOKS FROM THE BURNS ARCHIVE

2011	Sleeping Beauty III Memorial Photography: The Children
	Mirror, Mirror: Daguerreotypes from the Burns Collection
2009	Ophthalmology: A Photographic History 1840–1950 (4 Vol)
	News Art: Manipulated Photographs from the Burns Archive
2008	Deadly Intent, Crime & Punishment: Photographs from the Burns Archive
2007	Nephrology: A Photographic History 1840–1950 (4 Vol)
2006	Patients & Promise: A Photographic History of Mental and Mood Disorders (4 Vol)
	Geisha: A Photographic History 1872–1912
2005	Photographic History of Nineteenth Century Dermatology (4 Vol)
	Photographic History of Early Podiatry
2004	Oncology: Tumors & Treatment, A Photographic History 1845–1945 (4 Vol)
2003	Respiratory Disease: A Photographic History 1845–1945 (4 Vol)
2002	Sleeping Beauty II: Grief, Bereavement and the Family in Memorial Photography...
1999	A Mornings Work: Medical Photographs from The Burns Archive & Collection
1998	American Surgery: An Illustrated History
1995	Forgotten Marriage: The Painted Tintype & The Decorative Frame 1860–1910...
1994	Harm's Way: Lust & Madness, Murder & Mayhem
1993	The Face of Mercy: A Photographic History of Medicine at War
1991	Photographie et Médecine 1840–1880
1990	Sleeping Beauty: Memorial Photography in America
	The American Dentist: A Pictorial History
1987	Masterpieces of Medical Photography: Selections From The Burns Archive
1981/87	The Bristol® Gallery of Medical History (7 Volumes)
1983	Early Medical Photography in America: 1839–1883

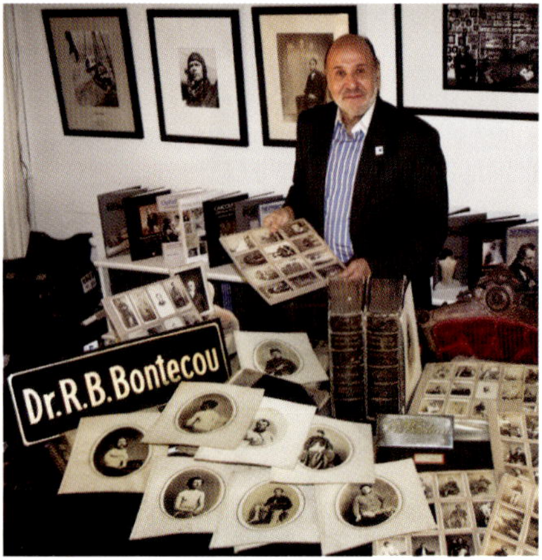

STANLEY B. BURNS, MD, a New York City ophthalmologist is an internationally distinguished author, curator, historian, collector, publisher, and archivist. In 1975 he began collecting historic photography and in 1977 founded The Burns Archive and began his writing and publishing career in order to share his discoveries. Dr. Burns' collection of vintage photographs (1840-1950) has been generally recognized as the most important private comprehensive collection of early photography. It has been showcased in numerous media venues worldwide. Artists, researchers and historians can access the over one million photographs.

"We should all be grateful to visionary leaders like Stanley Burns, MD, who not only take the initiative in preserving priceless historical photographic records but provide the context by which records of historical interest are understood to have importance and significance for contemporary health and medicine...just in time for the Sesquicentennial of the defining era of the American experience"

—Marc S. Micozzi, MD, PhD
Founding Director, National Museum of Health & Medicine (1986-1995)

INQUIRIES & BOOK ORDERS

Copies of *Shooting Soldiers...* can be ordered directly from The Burns Archive Press
140 East 38th Street, New York, New York 10016
Sleeping Beauty III Memorial Photography: The Children and other books in the 'Gem Series' can also be ordered directly from The Burns Archive Press.
www.burnsarchivepress.com www.burnsarchive.com

EXHIBITIONS

New York's Civil War Soldiers:
The Photographs of Dr. R. B. Bontecou. The Words of Walt Whitman.
April 28- August 1, 2011. Merchant's House Museum, 29 East Fourth Street, New York, NY 10003

R. B. Bontecou: Master Portraits of Civil War Soldiers
September 8- October 31, 2011. Robert Anderson Gallery, 24 West 57th Street, Suite 503, New York, NY 10019

Exhibitions of Burns Collection historic war, medical & memorial photographs are available as original prints for museums or as reproductions for public spaces in hospitals, universities, etc.

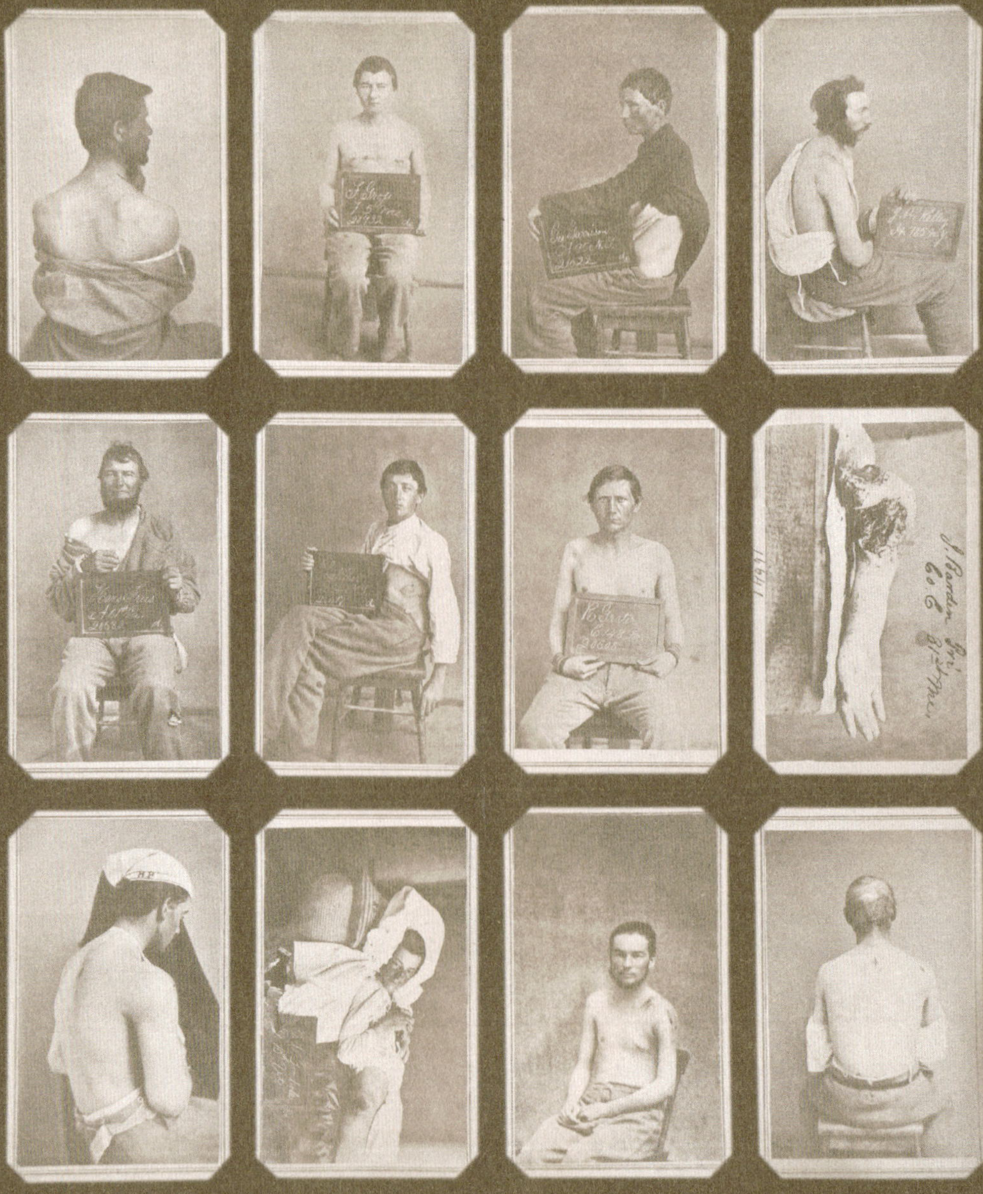